Second Edition

Strategies for Theory Construction in Nursing

Second Edition

Strategies for Theory Construction in Nursing

Lorraine Olszewski Walker, R.N., Ed.D.
Luci B. Johnson Centennial Professor
School of Nursing
The University of Texas at Austin
Austin, Texas

Kay Coalson Avant, R.N., Ph.D.
Associate Professor
School of Nursing
The University of Texas at Austin
Austin, Texas

APPLETON & LANGE
Norwalk, Connecticut/San Mateo, California

0-8385-8680-5

88 89 90 91 92 / 10 9 8 7 6 5 4 3 2 1

Prentice-Hall International (UK) Limited, *London*
Prentice-Hall of Australia Pty. Limited, *Sydney*
Prentice-Hall Canada, Inc., *Toronto*
Prentice-Hall Hispanoamericana, S.A., *Mexico*
Prentice-Hall of India Private Limited, *New Delhi*
Prentice-Hall of Japan, Inc., *Tokyo*
Simon & Schuster Asia Pte. Ltd., *Singapore*
Editora Prentice-Hall do Brasil Ltda., *Rio de Janeiro*
Prentice Hall, *Englewood Cliffs, New Jersey*

Library of Congress Cataloging-in-Publication Data

Walker, Lorraine Olszewski.
    Strategies for theory construction in nursing / Lorraine Olszewski
Walker, Kay Coalson Avant.—2nd ed.
        p. cm.
    Includes bibliographies and index.
    ISBN 0-8385-8680-5
    1. Nursing—Philosophy.   2. Theory (Philosophy)   I. Avant, Kay
Coalson.   II. Title.
    [DNLM: 1. Models, Theoretical—nurses' instruction.
2. Philosophy, Nursing.   WY 86 W181s]
    RT84.5.W34   1988
    610.73′01—dc19
    DNLM/DLC
    for Library of Congress   88-22254
                                                                                          CIP

Designer: Steven Byrum

Contents

Preface to the Second Edition

In this second edition we have tried to maintain the procedural focus of the first edition but elaborate on points in need of further clarification. We greatly appreciate the feedback received from users of the strategies in this regard; our efforts toward improvement would have been impossible without their work. In addition, we have updated references and made some format changes in this edition. To each strategies chapter we have added a section on using the results of the theoretic work generated. Also, introductory comments have been added to each of the five parts of the book to better orient readers.

Stepping back from the specific strategies, we note that major revolutions in the meta-theoretical and theoretical thinking of the discipline have transpired since the first edition was written. We have tried to sketch the richness and complexity of this thought in the introductory and concluding chapters of this second edition. In particular, we have completely rewritten Chapter 12 and added Chapter 13. Chapter 12 now focuses on theory testing and explicates the emerging theoretical foci in nursing literature. In Chapter 13 we give a brief overview of knowledge development and ways of knowing. However, our main purpose remains to elaborate strategies that may be useful in furthering the growth of nursing knowledge, specifically its theoretical base.

We are grateful to the staff of Appleton & Lange for their continued support during preparation of this second edition. We are indebted to Marion Kalstein Welch, Stuart Horton, and all the other editors and staff who were there at each step of the revision process. Also, we are deeply indebted to Jacqueline Fawcett, Ph.D., FAAN, for her penetrating critique of an earlier draft of this second edition. Finally, we are forever grateful to Charles Bollinger—dear friend, editor, and now antique dealer—for the seeds he planted that made this second edition possible.

We must acknowledge those who have supported the non-theoretical aspects of this work. To Misha, who tolerated invasion of her room, which housed the sacred computer, you are hereby extended a perpetual I.O.U. by your grateful mother. We are also appreciative of the many small ways in which other family members aided the preparation of this second edition.

L. W.
Austin, Texas
K. A.
Waco, Texas

Preface to the First Edition

Nursing as a profession has become very conscious of the need for theory development. As nursing has come of age, not only as a practice but also as a scholarly discipline, there has been increasing concern with delineating the theory base for nursing. There is no method text in nursing, however, that delineates approaches to theory construction.

This book, *Strategies for Theory Construction in Nursing*, is a method text on various approaches that may be used in constructing theory in nursing. Various approaches to theory construction are needed in order to accommodate factors pertinent to theory construction: (1) the presence or absence of research data about the subject matter of the theory, (2) the level of complexity of existing theoretical work in the area, (3) the congruence of extant theory and research findings, and (4) the particular perspective of each theory builder.

The approach taken in this book is pragmatic and procedural. Nine theory development strategies are presented with both general and specific directives and considerations relevant to each strategy. The aim of the authors is to avoid issues that are largely of philosophic interest and instead to focus on issues of direct concern to the theory builder. Procedures and strategies are presented in a detailed fashion with emphasis on "how to" considerations. Discussion of strategies and procedures aims at presenting material with clarity and illustrative examples. Explanations of strategies and procedures are provided along with limitations and advantages of these so that readers will find the book to be a generally self-contained reference on methods of theory construction. References are provided for readers who wish to pursue more technical or philosophical dimensions of strategies. Also, where available, other references on strategies are provided for readers who wish to consider several points of view on a strategy.

In this book we have done what some might find unthinkable: treating creative developments in a procedural fashion. We do not believe that theory construction is only a step-by-step procedure: Creativity on the part of the theorist is essential. We have tried, however, to demystify the intuitive processes that theorists use.

The pragmatic orientation selected by the authors has been chosen for several reasons. First, there is a wealth of philosophical and meta-theoretical discussion about nursing theory. To date, the meta-theoretical orientation has led to little substantive theory building. Second, the literature in the philosophy of science contains abundant discussions of philosophic and meta-theoretical issues pertinent to theory construction and theory verification. There is a gap, however, between these highly technical abstract works and the day-to-day activities of those interested in theory construction. It is this gap that we address.

The organization of this book reflects a developmental approach to theory. There are five parts. Part One gives a general overview of the state of the art in theory construction and an introduction to the framework and language used in the rest of the chapters. Parts Two, Three, and Four discuss the elements of theory construction: concept development, statement development, and theory development, respectively. There are three chapters in each part which reflect the three basic approaches we used: analysis, synthesis, and derivation. Each chapter concludes with one or more practice exercises with examples. Part Five discusses some final perspectives on theory construction that the authors felt were important for anyone to consider who plans active involvement in theory building.

Since this is intended as a methods text, the authors wish to clarify that both actual and hypothetical examples are used when illustrating strategies. The primary consideration in choosing examples was that they be useful in demonstrating the strategy to the reader. The scientific merits of the research and theory examples were necessarily a secondary consideration.

The authors wish to express their appreciation to Dr. Mary Walker for her unflagging encouragement and careful reading of our drafts. Her assistance, pertinent comments, and thoughtful suggestions helped immensely in completing this book. We are deeply grateful to Charles Bollinger, Senior Nursing Editor at Appleton-Century-Crofts, for his encouragement and support of this project from its inception to its completion. His excitement about it was infectious. Thanks must also be expressed to Mrs. Dot Martin for typing all our manuscripts with such speed, accuracy, and cheerful good humor. In addition, thanks must go to our families, Misha, Tim, Gayle, Samantha, and Celia, for their support and understanding. Finally, we cannot fail to mention Maggie Hank who catapulted us into this project.

Austin, Texas
Waco, Texas
December, 1981

PART I

Overview of Theory Development in Nursing

The two chapters in Part I provide background material to orient readers to the complex history and language of theory development in nursing. In Chapter 1 a brief overview is provided in which major past and present-day accomplishments in the field of nursing theory are noted. Four levels of nursing theory development (meta-theory, grand theory, middle-range theory, and practice theory) are proposed. Progress that has been made in each level is summarized. The logical distinction between the context of discovery and the context of justification is introduced and related to the need to develop strategies specific to the process of theory generation in nursing. Readers wishing to read primary source materials that have figured in the recent history of nursing meta-theory development will find many of these in Nicoll's (1986) book of readings. Reviews and summaries of substantive theories (or conceptual models) that have been important conceptual landmarks in nursing thought may be found in Fawcett (1984), Riehl and Roy (1980), and Fitzpatrick and Whall (1983) among others.

In Chapter 2 the basic vocabulary used in this book is presented and defined. The elements of theorizing (concepts, statements, and theories) are examined in terms of their definitions and relationships to each other and ultimately nursing science. The basic approaches to theory construction (analysis, synthesis, and derivation) are also in-

1

troduced in Chapter 2. Combining the three elements of theorizing with the three approaches results in nine distinct strategies for theory development: concept analysis, concept synthesis, concept derivation, statement analysis, statement synthesis, statement derivation, theory analysis, theory synthesis, and theory derivation. These form the substance of Parts II, III, and IV of this book. By carefully reading Chapter 2, readers should be able to make a preliminary decision about the strategy or strategies of theory development that are most suited to their needs and interests. Some readers may wish to confine their reading to only the strategies of direct relevance to their work. Others may wish to read all chapters on a given element, such as concepts, or on a particular approach, such as derivation. Lastly, some readers may simply prefer to read the book from beginning to end out of curiosity (or compulsion). To accommodate these varied reader preferences, we have written the nine strategy chapters so that they are independent of each other except where specifically cross-referenced.

REFERENCES

Fawcett J: Analysis and Evaluation of Conceptual Models of Nursing. Philadelphia: Davis, 1984.

Fitzpatrick JJ, Whall, AL: Conceptual Models of Nursing: Analysis and Application. Bowie, Md.: Brady, 1983.

Nicoll LH (ed.): Perspectives on Nursing Theory. Boston: Little, Brown, 1986.

Riehl JP, Roy, CR (eds.): Conceptual Models for Nursing Practice. 2d ed. New York: Appleton-Century-Crofts, 1980.

1

Theory Development
in Nursing:
Past and Present

INTRODUCTION

As nursing has come of age both as a profession and a scholarly discipline, there has been increasing concern with delineating its theory base. In 1978 Chinn and Jacobs asserted that "The development of theory is the most crucial task facing nursing today" (p. 1). What led to the interest in theory development? What progress has been made? What remains to be done? In this chapter, we will give attention to each of these questions. In so doing, we will mark off the differing levels of theory development and show how they relate to each other. This chapter closes by proposing that explicit methods of theory construction are needed and by relating creativity to such methods.

Interest in nursing theory development emerged for two reasons. First, nursing leaders saw theory development as a means of clearly establishing nursing as a profession. Theory development was inherent in the long-standing interest in defining nursing's body of knowledge. In a landmark paper early in this century, Flexner defined the characteristics of a profession. Included among Flexner's characteristics were the ideas that professions involve "intellectual operations" and "derive their raw material from science and learning" (quoted in Roberts, 1961, p. 101). Subsequent evaluations of nursing as a profession (Bixler and Bixler, 1945, 1959) specifically examined the extent to which nursing utilized and enlarged a "body of knowledge" for its practice. Thus, interest in the body of knowledge stemmed in part from the extrinsic value of the body of knowledge to the profession. As Donaldson and Crowley forcefully stated, ". . . the very survival of the profession may be at risk unless the discipline is defined" (1978, p. 114).

The second reason for interest in theory development was motivated by the intrinsic value of theory for nursing. Simply stated, growth and enrichment of theory were important to nursing as a field of study, that is, a discipline, regardless of other values it might have—political or economic. The intrinsic value of theory development was reflected in Bixler and Bixler's (1945) first criterion for a profession:

> A profession utilizes in its practice a well-defined and well-organized body of specialized knowledge which is on the intellectual level of . . . higher learning (p. 730).

Commitment to practice based on sound reliable knowledge is intrinsic to the idea of a profession and practice discipline. As the foundation for professional knowledge, theory provides a more complete picture for practice than factual knowledge alone. Theories include more aspects of practice and integrate them more fully than factual knowledge. In addition, theories that are well developed not only organize existing knowledge but also aid in making new and important discoveries to advance practice.

Recent reviews of the status of theory development in nursing have carried an optimistic tone. Fawcett (1983), for example, cited these four hallmarks of success in recent nursing theory development: "a metaparadigm for nursing, conceptual models for nursing, unique nursing theories, and nursing theories shared with other disciplines" (pp. 3–4). Similarly, in systematically reviewing nursing research articles from 1952 to 1980, Brown et al. (1984) noted a trend for authors "to lay explicit claim to a conceptual perspective" (pp. 28–29). Indeed over half the studies they reviewed were judged to contain explicit "conceptual perspectives" (p. 28).

LEVELS OF THEORY DEVELOPMENT

The desire to develop nursing's theory base has led to four levels of theory development literature. The first of these, *meta-theory*, focuses on philosophical and methodological questions related to the development of a theory base for nursing. The second, *grand nursing theories*, consists of global conceptual frameworks defining broad perspectives for practice and ways of looking at nursing phenomena based on these perspectives. Third, a less abstract level of theory, *middle-range theory*, is emerging to fill the gaps between grand nursing theories and nursing practice. Fourth, a practice-oriented level of theory, *practice theory*, also is advocated. In this fourth level of theory, prescriptions, or, more broadly, modalities, for practice are delineated. We will sketch out progress made on each of these four fronts. We will conclude the review of the levels of theory development in nursing by proposing a model that suggests how levels of theory development articulate with each other.

Meta-Theory
Meta-theory focuses on broad issues related to theory in nursing and does not generally produce any grand, middle-range, or practice theories. Issues debated at the level of meta-theory include but are not limited to (1) analyzing the purpose and kind of theory needed in nursing, (2) proposing and critiquing sources and methods of theory development in nursing, and (3) proposing the criteria most suited for evaluating theory in nursing. Threaded throughout the meta-theoretical literature are examinations of the meaning of nursing as a "practice discipline," that is, nursing as both science and profession. An inspection of Table 1.1 shows that meta-theory has received extensive attention in nursing. While some meta-theory is accompanied by companion efforts at the grand, middle-range, or practice levels, meta-theory has been largely a separate enterprise from these other levels of theory development. Because meta-theory represents many points of view about theory in nursing, it has not been consolidated into one unanimously accepted set of beliefs.

One of the major issues debated in early nursing meta-theory was the relationship of nursing theory to basic science theories (e.g., Wooldridge et al., 1968; Dickoff et al., 1968a, 1968b). More recently changes in philosophy of science itself have influenced nursing meta-theory. In a critical analysis of the philosophy of science embraced by nursing, Webster et al. (1981) have called for "exorcising the ghost of the Received View from nursing" (p. 26). They argue that nurses have uncritically clung to a number of doctrines about the nature of science that were prominent in the 1930s. Based on logical positivism, Received View doctrines include beliefs such as "theories are either true or false," "science has nothing to say about values," and "there is a single scientific method" (pp. 29–30). Jacox and Webster (1986) note the emergence of alternate philosophies of science, including historicism. They suggest that expanding the philosophical positions adopted in nursing should enrich both nursing theories and research.

In a related criticism, Silva and Rothbart (1984) also distinguish

TABLE 1.1. CHRONOLOGICAL LISTING OF SELECTED META-THEORY IN NURSING

Item	Source
The Process of Theory Development in Nursing	McKay, 1965
Symposium: Research—How Will Nursing Define It?	Research—How Will Nursing Define it? 1967
Behavioral Science, Social Practice, and the Nursing Profession	Wooldridge et al., 1968
Conference: The Nature of Science and Nursing	The Nature of Science and Nursing, 1968
Theory in a Practice Discipline	Dickoff et al., 1968a, 1968b
Symposium: Theory Development in Nursing	Theory Development in Nursing, 1968
First Nursing Theory Conference	Norris, 1969
Conference: The Nature of Science in Nursing	The Nature of Science in Nursing, 1969
Second Nursing Theory Conference	Norris, 1970
Third Nursing Theory Conference	Norris, 1971
Nursing as a Discipline	Walker, 1971a
Three-Part Series: Toward a Clearer Understanding of the Concept of Nursing Theory	Walker, 1971b; Commentary on Walker's "Toward . . . ," 1971; Walker, 1972
Symposium: Approaches to the Study of Nursing Questions and the Development of Nursing Science	Approaches to the Study of Nursing Questions and the Development of Nursing Science, 1972
Practice Oriented Theory	Advances in Nursing Science, 1978
Critique: Practice Theory	Beckstrand, 1978a, 1978b
Theory Development: What, Why, How?	National League for Nursing, 1978
Nursing Theory: Analysis, Application, Evaluation	Stevens, 1984
Nursing Theory and the Ghost of the Received View	Webster et al., 1981
The Nature of Theoretical Thinking in Nursing	Kim, 1983
An Analysis of Changing Trends in Philosophies of Science on Nursing Theory Development and Testing	Silva & Rothbart, 1984

between two major schools of philosophy of science, logical empiricism and historicism. They assert that these two schools differ in several fundamental dimensions, including the underlying conception of science. Logical empiricists emphasize understanding science as a product; historicists understand science from the standpoint of process (pp. 3–5). Similarly, logical empiricists and historicists differ in their ideas about the goals of philosophy of science and the components of science. Finally, Silva and Rothbart claim that logical empiricists assess scientific progress in terms of acceptance or rejection of theories, while historicists emphasize the number of scientific problems solved. While noting a stable commitment among nurses to logical empiricism, they acknowledge an emerging diversity in conceptual frameworks and research methods congruent with historicist perspectives.

As nurses have begun to rethink the meta-theoretical assumptions of the discipline, this rethinking has spawned a growing interest in alternate methodologies for nursing theory and research (e.g., Chinn, 1985; Gorenberg, 1983) in addition to more conventional scientific ones. Research methodologists increasingly differentiate the qualitative (Benoliel, 1984) and quantitative (Atwood, 1984) approaches. Although there are many ways to differentiate these two approaches, one of the most apparent differences is the use of statistical tests in drawing inferences within quantitative approaches. Indeed, some authors have proposed integrating both methods within research studies (Goodwin & Goodwin, 1984). The philosophical ferment about the nature and method of science, thus, has not only been the major focus of contemporary nursing meta-theory but has enlarged the approaches advocated for nursing research.

Readers who wish more detailed information about philosophy of science and nursing meta-theory will find excellent reviews in Stevenson and Woods (1986) and Suppe and Jacox (1985). For further readings in the philosophy of science, see the listing of additional readings at the close of this chapter.

We believe it is important to carefully consider the philosophical assumptions of present-day nursing theory development and research. We believe it is equally important to put into action principles that form the core of the self-corrective process of science. Central to this core is the idea of the scientific community: scholars who both work in independent laboratories or research sites and come together to learn from and examine each other's work. Two principles of operation that have traditionally been used within the scientific community are critique and replication. Thus, scientists actively seek and receive criticism of their work and attempt to reproduce findings independently. These principles serve several purposes, one of which is to maximize the likelihood that human and technical errors in scientific inference will be detected. Philosophical arguments about the Received and alternative views of science should not overshadow the need for critique and replication among working scientists. Rather, philosophical arguments that serve to clarify meaning and purpose need touchpoints with the operational principles of critique and replication guiding the work of nurse scientists.

Grand Nursing Theories

Grand theories are abstract and often have been proposed to give some broad perspective to the goals and structure of nursing practice. Not all grand theories are at the same level of abstraction or have exactly the same scope. On the whole, however, they are not limited enough to be classified as middle-range theories and have as their goal explicating a world view useful in understanding key concepts and principles within a nursing perspective. In a similar vein, Fawcett (1984b) used the term "conceptual models" for those "global ideas about the individuals, groups, situations, and events of interest to a discipline" (p. 2).

Grand theories have made an important contribution in conceptually sorting out nursing from the practice of medicine by demonstrating the presence of distinct nursing perspectives. While there may be some disagreement on what works constitute grand theories, Table 1.2 shows a representative listing of writings we would classify as grand theories in nursing.

The bulk of grand theories were developed from the early 1960s to the present. Peplau's (1952) exposition of nursing and its educative function with patients was an early example of grand nursing theory.

TABLE 1.2. REPRESENTATIVE GRAND NURSING THEORIES

Author	Date	Publication
Peplau	1952	Interpersonal Relations in Nursing
Orlando	1961	The Dynamic Nurse-Patient Relationship
Wiedenbach	1964	Clinical Nursing: A Helping Art
Henderson	1966	The Nature of Nursing
Levine	1967	The Four Conservation Principles of Nursing
Ujhely	1968	Determinants of the Nurse-Patient Relationship
Rogers	1970	An Introduction to the Theoretical Basis of Nursing
King	1971	Toward a Theory of Nursing
Orem	1971	Nursing: Concepts of Practice
Travelbee	1971	Interpersonal Aspects of Nursing
Neuman	1974	The Betty Neuman Health-Care Systems Model
Roy	1976	Introduction to Nursing: An Adaptation Model
Newman	1979	Toward a Theory of Health
Johnson	1980	The Behavioral System Model for Nursing
Parse	1981	Man-Living-Health
Watson	1985	Nursing: Human Science and Human Care
Newman	1986	Health as Expanding Consciousness

Grand theories in the 1960s, such as Orlando's *The Dynamic Nurse-Patient Relationship* (1961) and Wiedenbach's *Clinical Nursing: A Helping Art* (1964), focused on defining concepts centered in the nurse-patient relationship. For example, Wiedenbach emphasized the patient's "need-for-help" as distinct from nurse-defined patient needs. Orlando differentiated deliberative and automatic nursing actions. These two theorists' concepts helped nurses clarify and respond to patients' needs and behaviors. Later grand theories shifted from a focus on the nurse-patient relationship to more expansive concepts. For example, Rogers (1970) stressed a holistic perspective on the life process of "man." A multilevel systems model developed by King (1971) included the major concepts of perception, interpersonal relations, social systems, and health. Dorothy Johnson (1980) constructed a model of the client as a behavioral system composed of seven subsystems. Johnson's thinking was further reflected in Auger's (1976) behavioral systems model, which includes eight subsystems: the affiliative, dependency, ingestive, achievement, aggressive, eliminative, sexual, and restorative. While nurses might deal with medical and physiological data in the Johnson/Auger grand theories, the approach to these is distinctively a behavioral one. Recent grand theories have attempted to capture the phenomenological aspects of nursing. For example, Watson has adopted a "phenomenological-existential" orientation in her theory of human care (1985, p. x).

While the grand nursing theories have provided global perspectives for nursing practice, education, and research, these theories unfortunately are limited as they presently exist. By virtue of their generality and abstractness, most grand nursing theories are untestable in their present forms. While they may offer some general perspectives for practice or curriculum organization in nursing, by their very nature and purpose most of them would require major revision and expansion before testing would be possible. In revising and refining grand nursing theories, (1) vague terminology would need to be clarified, and (2) interrelationships between concepts in the theories themselves would need to be delineated with sufficient precision so that predictions can be made. In this line, several theorists have published revisions of their works in an effort to clarify and further elaborate them (e.g., see Roy & Roberts, 1981; King, 1981).

Still, most grand theories pose formidable problems for those wishing to test them. These problems relate to still another problem in grand theories: absent or weak linkages between terminology in the theories and their observational indicators. This is the point on which Suppe and Jacox (1985) critique the tests of the grand theory of Rogers: such tests are contingent on "auxiliary claims that provide most of the testable content" (p. 249). Fawcett and Downs (1986) are even more forceful as they assert that

> . . . [A] conceptual model [and/or grand theory] cannot be tested
> directly. Rather, the propositions of a conceptual model are tested
> indirectly through the empirical testing of theories that are de-
> rived or linked with the model. If the findings of theory-testing
> research support the theory, then it is likely that the conceptual
> model is credible (p. 89).

Thus it would appear that a layer of theorizing is needed between
grand theories and their empirical testing. This layer is congruent
with the idea of middle-range theory as proposed here.

Despite the complexity of most grand nursing theories, Silva
(1986) has identified 62 research studies that have used one or more
of these (Johnson, Orem, Roy, Rogers, and Newman) as a basis for
research. Unfortunately, only nine of the studies were found to adequately use the grand theories (termed "conceptual models" by Silva)
in theory testing. Silva partially attributed the imprecise use of theories in theory testing to the ambiguity of the concept of theory testing itself.

While some nurses have focused their work on the problems of
testing grand theories, others have directed their attention to areas
of commonality among grand theories (Flaskerud & Halloran, 1980).
Fawcett concluded, "A review of the literature on theory development
in nursing reveals a consensus about the central concepts of the
discipline—person, environment, health, and nursing" (1984a, p. 84).
As the broadest area of consensus within the nursing discipline,
these concepts constitute its metaparadigm (Fawcett, 1984b). In a
related vein, Meleis (1985) identified the following as "domain concepts": nursing client, transitions, interaction, nursing process, environment, nursing therapeutics, and health (p. 184). Small pockets of
work are beginning to emerge that link the four metaparadigm concepts to middle-range theorizing and research (see section in Chapter
12 on emerging theoretical foci in nursing). Others focus on only one
of the metaparadigm concepts, for example, Smith's (1981) analysis of
health's four models and Laffrey's (1986) generation of a measurement tool based on those four models.

Middle-Range Theories

Because of the difficulties inherent in testing grand theories, another
more workable level of theory development has been proposed (Jacox,
1974; See, 1981) and utilized in nursing: theories of the middle range.
Theories of this level contain limited numbers of variables and are
limited in scope as well. Because of these characteristics, middle-
range theories are testable, yet sufficiently general to still be scientifically interesting. Thus, middle-range theories share some of the
conceptual economy of grand theories but also provide the specificity

needed for usefulness in research and practice. The work of Caplan and others presented in Chapter 10 is an example of theory aimed at the middle range. Also, Fawcett (1986) has proposed that the list of alphabetically arranged nursing diagnoses developed by the North American Nursing Diagnosis Association is a middle-range theory (p. 397).

In order to identify middle-range theories that are in use within nursing, we conducted an informal content analysis of six recent successive issues of both *Nursing Research* and *Research in Nursing and Health*. The clearest and most frequently used example of middle-range theory we encountered was the health belief model (see Massey, 1986; Champion, 1985; Kviz et al., 1985). Others we identified but that were expressed less clearly or directly in the research were theories of coping, maternal role attainment, and maternal attachment, among others. (In Chapter 12 we present the results of that content analysis in more detail as we propose emerging theoretical foci of nursing investigations.)

Practice Theory

One outgrowth of nursing meta-theory has been the idea of practice theory (Wooldridge et al., 1968; Dickoff et al., 1968a). In describing practice theory, Jacox (1974) provided the following succinct description:

> It is theory that says given this nursing goal (producing some desired change or effect in the patient's condition), these are the actions the nurse must take to meet the goal (produce the change). For example, a nursing goal may be to prevent a postoperative patient from becoming hyponatremic. Nursing practice theory states that, to prevent hyponatremia, a particular set of actions must be taken (p. 10).

The essence of practice theory is a desired goal and prescriptions for action to achieve the goal.

Within the Dickoff et al. proposal for practice theory, progress through four phases of theorizing was supposed to lead to the theory base for nursing practice. These phases included factor-isolating, factor-relating, situation-relating, and situation-producing or practice theory. These four phases roughly paralleled the acts of description, explanation, prediction, and control. If a practice theory were separated from its base in situation-relating (predictive) theory, readers can readily see that the remaining prescriptions and goal constitute a rather generous extension of the usual meaning of "theory." Some readers may simply wish to drop the word "theory" for this reason and think of practice theory as "nursing practices." Where practices are defined as specification of a desired goal and prescriptions for action to achieve that goal, we see little distinction between practices and practice theory as we have discussed them here (Beckstrand, 1978a, 1978b).

We note special progress that has been made at the level of developing practices. We find the Conduct and Utilization of Research in Nursing project of special interest (Haller et al., 1979). In this project research-based knowledge is transferred into "protocols for nursing practice" (p. 45). Among the practice protocols studied were (1) sensation information: distress, (2) intravenous cannula change regimen, (3) prevention of decubiti by means of small shifts of body weight, and (4) deliberate nursing: pain reduction. Further, two recently released books devoted to nursing interventions hold special promise for expanding the foundations of nursing practices (Snyder, 1985; Bulechek & McCloskey, 1985).

Linkages Among Levels of Theory Development

From reading the preceding sections it should be clear that one cannot reasonably ask at what level nursing theory development should occur: Work has and is being done at each level. A more fitting question is, how are the levels of theory development related to each other? In Figure 1.1 we propose a model of the linkages between and among the four levels of theory development. Meta-theory, through analysis of issues about nursing theory, clarifies the methodology and roles of each level of theory development in a practice discipline. In turn, each level of theory provides material for further analysis and clarification at the level of meta-theory. Grand nursing theories by their global perspectives serve as guides and heuristics for the phenomena of special concern at the middle-range level of theory. For example, Fawcett (1978) used the work of Rogers (1970) to develop a descriptive theory of body image and identification in pregnant coup-

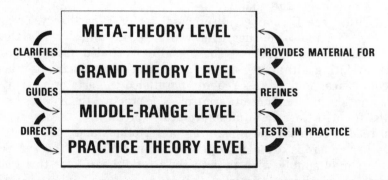

Figure 1.1. Linkages Among Levels of Theory Development

les. Further, middle-range theories, as they are tested in reality, become reference points for further refining grand nursing theories to which they may be connected (see an example of this connection in Gill & Atwood, 1981). Middle-range theories also direct the prescriptions of practice theories aimed at concrete goal attainments. Finally, practice theory, which is constructed from scientifically based propositions about reality, tests (if only indirectly) the empirical validity of those propositions as practices are incorporated in patient care. Those propositions most relevant to practice theory are likely to come from middle-range theories because their language is more easily tied to concrete situations.

Despite the variety of linkages between the levels of theory development, none of them directly represent actual methods or strategies for theory construction. While meta-theory, for instance, illuminates important issues to consider in a developing profession and science, a gap between meta-theory and methods for actual production of scientific theory exists. Similarly the Dickoff et al. proposal for practice theory does not provide clear and specific procedures to use in constructing a practice theory. Obviously something more is needed if nursing is to move effectively toward the construction of its theory base.

NEED FOR NEW DIRECTIONS
IN THEORY BUILDING

In this section, we propose two ingredients we believe will facilitate the development of nursing theory. These ingredients are focused on producing theory at the grand and middle-range levels of generality. We believe that theory development focused at these levels can be facilitated by (1) carefully distinguishing between the context of discovery and the context of justification in constructing theory, and (2) delineating specific strategies and procedures for theory building. While these ingredients may not be new in themselves, we believe that persistent and committed attention to them is.

Contexts of Discovery and Justification
The construction of theory is distinct from the evaluation of theory. Rudner (1966) used the terms "context of discovery" and "context of justification" respectively to differentiate between the processes of developing and evaluating ideas. The generation of theory involves initially constructing theory without immediate knowledge of its usefulness or accuracy. Theory evaluation in turn serves to highlight the strengths and weaknesses of theory by examining the outcomes of

theory testing in reality and by comparing the theory with other criteria, such as logical consistency. Prematurely imposing the standards and methods used in theory evaluation upon theory generation can lead to rejection of a promising theory and stifling of the creative process. Further, criticizing the methods or origins from which a theory has been developed because these do not conform to those used in theory evaluation is equally dangerous. While a well-developed theory should be expected to pass review by rigorous standards for theory evaluation, these same standards may not be appropriate for generating theory. For example, small samples or case studies might be employed in developing a theory of early adjustment to parenthood. In testing and evaluating the theory, however, these same data might be judged to be inadequate in size and objectivity. However, disregarding these data during theory generation would be imprudent because valuable insights may be lost. Bearing in mind the difference between discovery and evaluation frees the theory developer of unnecessary restrictions that might be useful in the context of justification but obstructive in the context of discovery.

Methods of Theory Construction
Clear and explicit methods of theory construction in nursing are needed. To date, the methods for developing the theory base in nursing have not been delineated in any complete manner. Methodologies currently available in other disciplines, such as sociology (Hage, 1972), have not been translated into a nursing context. In recognition of this need, we have written this methods book. In the chapters that follow, methods for constructing theory are described. The methods are presented with emphasis on theory construction, not evaluation. [Readers interested in theory evaluation are referred to the works of Ellis (1968), Hardy (1978), and Stevens (1984).] The methods, while equally suited to grand theories or middle-range theories, are generally presented from the vantage point of the latter.

Theory Construction and Creativity
There are both proponents and opponents of organized approaches to theory construction. We, of course, believe that using explicit approaches to theory construction can facilitate development of theory. Others would argue otherwise. Opponents see theory development as a non-rule-governed activity. Successful theorizing is, for them, based on the creativity of the theorist. In this line, Hempel (1966, p. 15) argued that there are no rules for mechanically deriving hypotheses or theories from data. We would of course agree with this. We do not propose to present a set of iron-clad rules for theory construction in

this book. What we do propose is a comprehensive set of strategies that can augment the intuitive processes that theorists already use in forming concepts, statements, and theories. We see strategies as guidelines for activities. As guidelines, strategies give theorists their bearings but do not remove the burden of creative work from the theorist.

REFERENCES

Approaches to the study of nursing questions and the development of nursing science. Nurs Res 21: 484–517, 1972.

Atwood JR: Advancing nursing science: Quantitative approaches. West J Nurs Res 6(3): 9–15, 1984.

Auger JR: Behavioral Systems and Nursing. Englewood Cliffs, N. J.: Prentice-Hall, 1976.

Beckstrand J: The need for a practice theory as indicated by the knowledge used in the conduct of practice. Res Nurs Health 1: 175–179, 1978a.

Beckstrand J: The notion of a practice theory and the relationship of scientific and ethical knowledge to practice. Res Nurs Health 1: 131–136, 1978b.

Benoliel JQ: Advancing nursing science: Qualitative approaches. West J Nurs Res 6(3): 1–8, 1984.

Bixler G, Bixler RW: The professional status of nursing. Amer J Nurs 45: 730–735, 1945.

Bixler G, Bixler RW: The professional status of nursing. Amer J Nurs 59: 1142–1147, 1959.

Brown JS, Tanner CA, Padrick KP: Nursing's search for scientific knowledge. Nurs Res 33: 26–32, 1984.

Bulechek GM, McCloskey JC (eds.): Nursing Interventions: Treatments for Nursing Diagnoses. Philadelphia: Saunders, 1985.

Champion VL: Use of the health belief model in determining frequency of breast self-examination. Res Nurs Health 8: 373–379, 1985.

Chinn PL: Debunking myths in nursing theory and research. Image 17: 45–49, 1985.

Chinn PL, Jacobs MK: A model for theory development in nursing. Adv Nurs Sci 1(1): 1–11, 1978.

Commentary on Walker's "Toward a clearer understanding of the concept of nursing theory." Nurs Res 20: 493–502, 1971.

Dickoff J, James P, Wiedenbach E: Theory in a practice discipline, Part I. Nurs Res 17: 415–435, 1968a.

Dickoff J, James P, Wiedenbach E: Theory in a practice discipline, Part II. Nurs Res 17: 545–554, 1968b.

Donaldson SK, Crowley DM: The discipline of nursing. Nurs Outlook 26: 113–120, 1978.

Ellis R: Characteristics of significant theories. Nurs Res 17: 217–222, 1968.

Fawcett J: The "what" of theory development. In Theory Development: What, Why, How? New York: National League for Nursing, 1978.

Fawcett J: Hallmarks of success in nursing theory development. In (PL Chinn, ed.), Advances in Nursing Theory Development. Rockville, MD: Aspen, 1983.

Fawcett J: The metaparadigm of nursing: Present status and future refinements. Image 16: 84–87, 1984a.

Fawcett J: Analysis and Evaluation of Conceptual Models of Nursing. Philadelphia: Davis, 1984b.

Fawcett J: Guest editorial: Conceptual models of nursing, nursing diagnosis, and nursing theory development. West J Nurs Res 8: 397–399, 1986.

Fawcett J, Downs F: The Relationship of Theory and Research, Norwalk, Conn.: Appleton-Century-Crofts, 1986.

Flaskerud JH, Halloran EJ: Areas of agreement in nursing theory development. Adv Nurs Sci 3(1): 1–7, 1980.

Gill BP, Atwood JR: Reciprocy and helicy used to relate mEGF and wound healing. Nurs Res 30: 68–72, 1981.

Goodwin LD, Goodwin WL: Qualitative vs. quantitative research or qualitative and quantitative research? Nurs Res 33: 378–380, 1984.

Gorenberg B: The research tradition of nursing: An emerging issue. Nurs Res 32: 347–349, 1983.

Hage J: Techniques and Problems of Theory Construction in Sociology. New York: Wiley, 1972.

Haller KB, Reynolds MA, Horsley JA: Developing research-based innovation protocols: Process, criteria, and issues. Res Nurs Health 2: 45–51, 1979.

Hardy ME: Perspectives on nursing theory. Adv Nurs Sci 1: 37–48, 1978.

Hempel CG: Philosophy of Natural Science. Englewood Cliffs, N. J.: Prentice-Hall, 1966.

Henderson V: The Nature of Nursing. New York: Macmillan, 1966.

Jacox A: Theory construction in nursing: An overview. Nurs Res 23: 4–13, 1974.

Jacox AK, Webster G: Competing theories of science. In (LH Nicoll, ed.), Perspectives on Nursing Theory. Boston: Little, Brown, 1986.

Johnson, DE: The behavioral system model for nursing. In (JP Riehl & C Roy, eds.), Conceptual Models for Nursing Practice. 2d ed. New York: Appleton-Century-Crofts, 1980.

Kim HS: The Nature of Theoretical Thinking in Nursing. Norwalk, Conn.: Appleton-Century-Crofts, 1983.

King I: Toward a Theory of Nursing. New York: Wiley, 1971.

King I: A Theory for Nursing: Systems, Concepts, Process. New York: Wiley, 1981.

Kviz FJ, Dawkins CE, Erum NE: Mothers' health beliefs and use of well-baby services among a high-risk population. Res Nurs Health 8: 381–387, 1985.

Laffrey SC: Development of a health conception scale. Res Nurs Health 9: 107–113, 1986.

Levine M: The four conservation principles of nursing. Nurs Forum 6(1): 45–59, 1967.

Massey V: Perceived susceptibility to breast cancer and practice of breast self-examination. Nurs Res 35: 183–185, 1986.

McKay RP: The Process of Theory Development in Nursing. Doctoral dissertation. New York: Columbia Univ., 1965.

Meleis AI: Theoretical Nursing. Philadelphia: Lippincott, 1985.

National League for Nursing. Theory Development: What, Why, How? New York: National League for Nursing, 1978.

The Nature of Science and Nursing: Nurs Res 17: 484–512, 1968.

The Nature of Science in Nursing. Nurs Res 18: 388–411, 1969.

Neuman B: The Betty Neuman health-care systems model: A total person approach to patient problems. In (JP Riehl & C Roy, eds.), Conceptual

Models for Nursing Practice. New York: Appleton-Century-Crofts, 1974.

Newman MA: Toward a theory of health. Chapter 6. In Theory Development in Nursing. Philadelphia: Davis, 1979.

Newman MA: Health as Expanding Consciousness. St. Louis: Mosby, 1986.

Norris CM (ed.): Proceedings of the First Nursing Theory Conference. Kansas City: Univ. of Kansas Medical Center, Dept. of Nursing, 1969.

Norris CM (ed.): Proceedings of the Second Nursing Theory Conference. Kansas City: Univ. of Kansas Medical Center, Dept. of Nursing, 1970.

Norris CM (ed.): Proceedings of the Third Nursing Theory Conference. Kansas City: Univ. of Kansas Medical Center, Dept. of Nursing, 1971.

Orem D: Nursing: Concepts of Practice. New York: McGraw-Hill, 1971.

Orlando IJ: The Dynamic Nurse-Patient Relationship. New York: Putnam, 1961.

Parse RR: Man-Living-Health: A Theory of Nursing. New York: Wiley, 1981.

Peplau HE: Interpersonal Relations in Nursing. New York: Putnam, 1952.

Practice Oriented Theory, Part I. Adv Nurs Sci 1(1): 1–95, 1978.

Research—How will nursing define it? Nurs Res 16: 108–129, 1967.

Roberts MA: American Nursing: History and Interpretation. New York: Macmillan, 1961, 101.

Rogers ME: An Introduction to the Theoretical Basis of Nursing. Philadelphia: Davis, 1970.

Roy C: Introduction to Nursing: An Adaptation Model. Englewood Cliffs, N.J.: Prentice-Hall, 1976.

Roy C, Roberts SL: Theory Construction in Nursing: An Adaptation Model. Englewood Cliffs, N.J.: Prentice-Hall, 1981.

Rudner R: Philosophy of Social Science. Englewood Cliffs, N.J.: Prentice-Hall, 1966.

See EM: Theories of middling-range generality in the development of nursing theory. Paper presented at the meeting of the Nursing Theory Think Tank, Denver, 1981.

Silva MC: Research testing nursing theory: State of the art. Adv Nurs Sci 9(1): 1–11, 1986.

Silva MC, Rothbart D: An analysis of changing trends in philosophies of science in nursing theory development and testing. Adv Nurs Sci 6(2): 1–13, 1984.

Smith JA: The idea of health: A philosophic inquiry. Adv Nurs Sci 3(3): 43–50, 1981.

Snyder M: Independent Nursing Interventions. New York: Wiley, 1985.

Stevens BJ: Nursing Theory: Analysis, Application, Evaluation. 2d ed. Boston: Little, Brown, 1984.

Stevenson JS, Woods NF: Nursing science and contemporary science: Emerging paradigms. In (GE Sorensen, ed.), Setting the Agenda for the Year 2000. Kansas City, Mo.: American Academy of Nursing, 1986.

Suppe F, Jacox AK: Philosophy of science and the development of nursing theory. In (HH Werley & JJ Fitzpatrick, eds.), Annual Review of Nursing Research 3: 241–267, 1985.

Theory Development in Nursing. Nurs Res 17: 196–227, 1968.

Travelbee J: Interpersonal Aspects of Nursing. Philadelphia: Davis, 1971.

Ujhely G: Determinants of the Nurse-Patient Relationship. New York: Springer, 1968.

Walker LO: Nursing as a Discipline. Doctoral dissertation. Bloomington, Ind.: Indiana Univ., 1971a.

Walker LO: Toward a clearer understanding of the concept of nursing theory. Nurs Res 20: 428–435, 1971b.

Walker LO: Rejoinder to commentary: Toward a clearer understanding of the concept of nursing theory. Nurs Res 21: 59–62, 1972.

Watson J: Nursing: Human Science and Human Care. Norwalk, Conn.: Appleton-Century-Crofts, 1985.

Webster G, Jacox A, Baldwin B: Nursing theory and the ghost of the received view. In (JC McCloskey & HK Grace, eds.), Current Issues in Nursing. Boston: Blackwell, 1981.

Wiedenbach E: Clinical Nursing: A Helping Art. New York: Springer, 1964.

Wooldridge P, Skipper JK, Leonard RC: Behavioral Science, Social Practice, and the Nursing Profession. Cleveland: Case Western Reserve, 1968.

ADDITIONAL READINGS IN PHILOSOPHY OF SCIENCE

Introductory readings are preceded by an *.

Aronson JL: A Realist Philosophy of Science. London: Macmillan, 1984.

Bhaskar R: A Realist Theory of Science. Atlantic Highlands, N.J.: Humanities Press, 1978.

*Cook TD, Campbell DT: Quasi-Experimentation: Design & Analysis Issues for Field Settings. Boston: Houghton Mifflin, 1979, 1–36.

Feyerabend P: Against Method: Outline of an Anarchistic Theory of Knowledge. London: Verso, 1975.

Glymour C: Theory and Evidence. Princeton, N.J.: Princeton Univ. Press, 1980.

Grunfeld J: Science and Values. Amsterdam: B. R. Gruner B. V., 1973.

Harre R: Varieties of Realism: A Rationale for the Natural Sciences. New York: Basil Blackwell, 1986.

Komesaroff PA: Objectivity, Science and Society: Interpreting Nature and Society in the Age of the Crisis of Science. New York: Routledge & Kegan Paul, 1986.

Kuhn TS: The Structure of Scientific Revolutions. 2d ed. Chicago: Univ. of Chicago Press, 1970.

Lakatos I, Musgrave A (eds.): Criticism and the Growth of Knowledge. London: Cambridge Univ. Press, 1970.

Lamb D, Easton SM: Multiple Discovery: The Pattern of Scientific Progress. England: Avebury, 1984.

Laudan L: Progress and Its Problems: Toward a Theory of Scientific Growth. Berkeley, Calif.: Univ. of California Press, 1977.

Michalos AC (ed.): Philosophical Problems of Science & Technology. Boston: Allyn & Bacon, 1974.

Popper KR: Conjectures and Refutations: The Growth of Scientific Knowledge. New York: Harper & Row, 1965.

*Radnitzky G: Contemporary Schools of Metascience. Chicago: Henry Regnery, 1973.

2

Introduction to Elements, Approaches, and Strategies of Theory Development

INTRODUCTION

Clear definitions, careful observation, and hard thinking are the best tools of the potential theory builder. To discuss theory building in a meaningful way, we must have some basic understanding among ourselves about the meanings of certain terms that will be used throughout the following chapters. This chapter is devoted to explaining these basic terms and demonstrating, in a general way, how they are related to each other. It is very important to be sure that agreement on meanings of terms is established at the beginning of our discussion.

There are three basic elements of theory building and three basic approaches for building these elements that will occupy our attention in this chapter. The three elements are concepts, statements, and theories. The three approaches are analysis, synthesis, and derivation. We will discuss the basic elements first and the approaches later in this chapter. We will demonstrate the relationship of the elements to the approaches in the strategy selection section of the chapter.

ELEMENTS OF THEORY BUILDING

Concepts

The basic building blocks of theory are concepts (Hardy, 1974). A *concept* is a mental image of a phenomenon; an idea or a construct in the mind about a thing or an action. It is *not* the thing or action, only the image of it. Concept formation begins in infancy, for concepts help us categorize or organize our environmental stimuli. Concepts help us identify how our experiences are similar or equivalent by categorizing all the things that are alike about them. Concept formation is thus a very efficient way of learning.

Concepts can be primitive, concrete, or abstract. Primitive concepts are those that have a common shared meaning among all individuals in a culture. For instance, a primitive concept like the color "blue" cannot be defined other than by giving examples of "blue" and "not blue." Concrete concepts are those that can be defined by primitive concepts, are limited by time and space, and are observable in reality. Abstract concepts are also capable of being defined by primitive or concrete concepts, but they are independent of time and space (Reynolds, 1971). The concept of "temperature," for instance, is abstract, while the concept of "temperature in Kansas City" is concrete because it is dependent on a specific place.

Concepts are expressed by means of language. The language "labels," or words, we use to express a concept are useful in communicating our ideas to other people. These "labels" are *not* the concept, they are only our way of communicating our concept. Thus the "labels," or words, may be found inadequate at times when we are attempting to get someone to understand our ideas or are trying to define something completely new.

Concepts are often referred to as "variables." This is easy to do, because when concepts can be defined operationally they may be used in research and are thus considered "variables" in the design. Nevertheless, they remain "concepts" when considered in the context of theory building.

Concepts allow us to classify our experiences in a meaningful way both to ourselves and others. They prove even *more* useful, however, when relationships can be drawn between two or more concepts. When such a relationship has been observed, it is expressed as a statement.

Statements

A *statement* is an extremely important ingredient in any attempt to build a scientific body of knowledge. It must be formulated before explanations or predictions can be made. A statement, in the context of theory building, can occur in two forms, relational statements and nonrelational statements. A relational statement declares a relationship of some kind between two or more concepts. A nonrelational statement may be either an existence statement that asserts the existence of the concept (Reynolds, 1971), or a definition, either theoretical or operational.

Relational statements either assert association (correlation) or causality (Reynolds, 1971). Associational statements are simply those that state which concepts occur together. They may even state in which direction the association occurs, for example, positively, negatively, or none. A positive association implies that as one concept occurs or changes the other concept occurs or changes in the same direction. For example, a positive association is demonstrated by the statement "Palmar sweating increases as anxiety increases." A negative association implies that as one concept occurs or changes the other concept occurs or changes in the opposite direction. For example, the statement "As maternal anxiety increases, maternal attachment behavior decreases" is a negative association. The "none" relationship implies that the occurrence of one concept tells us nothing about the occurrence of the other concept.

Causal statements demonstrate a cause-and-effect relationship. The concept that causes the change in the other concept may be referred to in research as the independent variable and the concept that is changed or affected, the dependent variable. An example of a causal statement might be "The application of undiluted bleach (NaOH) to a colored cotton cloth will cause the color in the cloth to fade."

Nonrelational statements serve as adjuncts to relational statements. They are the way by which the theorist clarifies meanings in the theory. Existence statements are usually simple statements of assertion about a concept. They are especially useful when the theorist is dealing with highly abstract material. For instance, the assertion "There is a phenomenon known as maternal attachment" is an existence statement. If little was known about the existence of such a phenomenon, it would be helpful to a reader for the theorist to thus label his or her concept and claim its existence as a starting place in the theory.

Theoretical definitions are the means by which the theorist introduces the reader to the critical attributes of each concept. These definitions are usually abstract and may not be measurable. Operational definitions reflect the theoretical definitions but they must have the measurement specifications included (Hardy, 1974). Theoretical and operational definitions are critical in theory building. Without them there is no way to test and thus validate the theory in the "real world."

Theories

A theory is an internally consistent group of relational statements (concepts, definitions, and propositions) that presents a systematic view about a phenomenon and that is useful for description, explanation, prediction, and control. A theory, by virtue of its predictive potential, is the primary means of meeting the goals of the nursing profession concerned with a clearly defined body of knowledge. Theory is usually constructed to express a new idea or a new insight into the nature of a phenomenon of interest.

Each of the four functions of theory—description, explanation, prediction, and control—represents a different phase of theory development. The ideal theory would do all these things well. However, we do not have an ideal theory in any discipline. Because science is evolutionary and because the human organism is intrinsically fallible, theories are always changing. At any point in time, the various theories in a discipline may be found at all stages of development. Some theories are specifically designed as explanations, such as the theory of evolution, without any intention of predictability. Others are designed specifically to yield predictability but do not provide control. For example, earthquakes may be predicted but not yet controlled. We ought not despair at this apparently imperfect world of theory building. Scientific thought grows through a self-correcting process. The submission of one's ideas to the critique and analysis of one's colleagues leads to a phenomenon of revision, validation, and extension of a given theory.

In theory building, theories are often graphically represented by means of models. As Baltes et al. have noted, a model is "any device used to represent something other than itself" (1977, p. 17). The parts of a model should correspond to, or be isomorphic to, the parts of the theory they represent (Brodbeck, 1968, p. 583). A model may be drawn mathematically, as an equation for instance, or it may be drawn schematically using symbols and arrows. A mathematical model might look something like this:

$$Y = {}_{a_1}X^{(1)} + {}_{a_2}X^{(2)} + {}_{a_3}X^{(3)} + E$$

In this equation Y represents a dependent criterion variable, X represents an independent (predictor) variable, each a represents the mathematical weighting applied to the respective X's, and E represents an error term (unexplained variance). A schematic model might look more like Figure 2.1.

Models can be developed either pretheoretically or posttheoretically. The pretheoretical model acts either as a heuristic device or as an attempt by the theorist to discover missing linkages in early

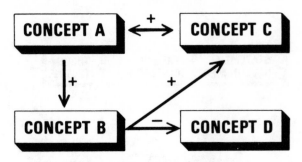

Figure 2.1. Schematic Model

theorizing. The posttheoretical model is developed after the theory and to lay bare the internal and formal structure of the theory—the system of interrelationships of the concepts.

In nursing, the term "model" has still another specialized meaning: "the image of the entire field and concepts of all its major units—the goal, patiency, and so forth" (Riehl & Roy, 1980, p. 7). For the purposes of this book, the term *model*, however, will be used only in its mathematical or schematic sense. This stipulated usage of "model" is necessary to quantify and clarify the relationships between concepts in any theoretical work. For further clarification of levels and types of models, see the Additional Readings section at the end of this chapter.

INTERRELATEDNESS OF ELEMENTS

Because theories encompass both concepts and statements, theory development frequently begins at the level of these latter two elements. For example, in the complete process of theory development, a theorist might start with concept development. As this is accomplished, the goals of statement development and ultimately theory development would be pursued. Only when one has a unified account of a set of relationships, as theories provide, can the goals of prediction and explanation in science be achieved (Hempel, 1966). Theories need, of course, to be tested through research and practice. Testing may in turn highlight areas within theories where revision is needed. At this point the process of theory development is begun again. These phases of theory development are graphically shown in Figure 2.2. Thus, theory development, research, and practice are part of the larger process of the scientific development of a discipline, not separate processes that are ends in themselves. While this book will

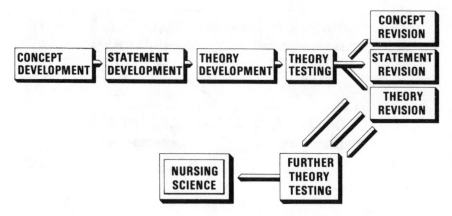

Figure 2.2. Phases in the Development of Nursing Science

focus on theory development in nursing, readers should keep in mind the interdependence of theory with research and practice.

APPROACHES TO THEORY BUILDING

The three basic approaches to theory building we use in this book are analysis, synthesis, and derivation. While a theory builder may move back and forth among these approaches, we will present them separately to aid the beginner in getting a better picture of each one.

Analysis

In *analysis*, one clarifies, refines, or sharpens concepts, statements, or theories. Analysis is especially useful in areas in which there is an existing body of theoretical literature. In this approach the theorist dissects a whole into its component parts so they can be better understood (Bloom, 1956, p. 205). In addition, the theorist examines the relationship of each of the parts to each of the other parts and to the whole. For example, the concept of empathy occurs frequently in the nursing literature. If there are competing or inconsistent points of view about empathy, then an analysis of this concept can help clarify the use, nature, and properties of the concept.

Synthesis

Synthesis, in contrast, combines isolated pieces of information that are as yet theoretically unconnected (Bloom, 1956, p. 206). In synthesis, information based on observation is used to construct a new concept, a new statement, or a new theory. Synthesis works well where a theorist is collecting data or trying to interpret data without an explicit theoretical framework. Much descriptive clinical research consists of collecting large amounts of data in the hope of sifting out important factors and relationships. Synthesis can aid in this sifting process. For example, nurses in school settings might use academic and family information to try to identify factors associated with teenage drug abuse or pregnancy.

Derivation

Finally, *derivation* employs analogy or metaphor in transposing and redefining a concept, statement, or theory from one context to another. Our strategy of derivation is heavily influenced by the work of Maccia and Maccia (1966) on educational theory models. This third approach to theory building can be applied to areas in which no theory base exists. Derivation may also be used in fields in which there are existing theories that have become outmoded and new innovative perspectives are needed. Derivation provides a means of theory building through shifting the terminology or the structure from one field or context to another. For example, one might take a concept from chemistry, such as chemical equilibrium, and, by analogy, use it to derive a description of how information exchange occurs within a group of professionals.

Strategy Selection

To further define the three approaches to theory building, we have superimposed them on the three elements of theory. Nine *strategies* for theory building result from this cross-classification of elements and approaches. The strategies and their specific uses in theory building are presented in Table 2.1. By carefully determining the elements of theory desired and the nature of available literature and information on a topic, the theorist may use Table 2.1 as a guide to strategy selection. To determine a suitable theory-building strategy, first of all, the theory builder must be clear about his or her area of interest. Next a theorist must decide whether to focus on concepts, statements, or the overall theory. This will depend on the quality of concept, statement, and theory development that already exists in the area of interest. Theorists may ask themselves several questions to determine which *element* best fits their needs.

1. What is the existing extent of theory development on the topic of interest?
2. How adequate is the existing theory development?
3. In which element is the available theory the weakest: concepts, statements, or the overall theory?

**TABLE 2.1. STRATEGIES OF THEORY BUILDING
RESULTING FROM CROSS-CLASSIFICATION OF
ELEMENTS OF THEORY WITH APPROACHES TO
THEORY BUILDING**

Elements of Theory	Approaches to Theory Building		
	Analysis	*Synthesis*	*Derivation*
Concept	Strategy: Concept analysis (Ch. 3)	Strategy: Concept synthesis (Ch. 4)	Strategy: Concept derivation (Ch. 5)
	Use: To clarify or refine an existing concept.	Use: To extract or pull together concept(s) from a body of data or set of observations.	Use: To shift and redefine concept(s) from one field to another.
Statement	Strategy: Statement analysis (Ch. 6)	Strategy: Statement synthesis (Ch. 7)	Strategy: Statement derivation (Ch. 8)
	Use: To clarify or refine an existing body of statements.	Use: To extract or pull together one or more statements from a body of data or set of observations.	Use: To shift and reformulate the content or structure of statements from one field to another.
Theory or *Theoretical Model*	Strategy: Theory analysis (Ch. 9)	Strategy: Theory synthesis (Ch. 10)	Strategy: Theory derivation (Ch. 11)
	Use: To clarify or refine an existing theory.	Use: To pull together a theory from a body of data, set of observations, or set of empirical statements.	Use: To shift and reformulate the content or structure of theories from one field to another.

4. What do review articles suggest about the kind of theory development needed next on the topic?

5. What is my personal judgment about the element of theory development that would be the most productive for me to pursue now on my topic of interest?

Carefully consider these questions. Your answers should help you clarify where you should begin theory building: with concepts, statements, or the whole theory.

The extent and type of literature and data available on a topic provide a basis for selecting the *approach* to be used. Here the theorist may ask another set of questions.

1. Is there any existing literature on the topic?
2. If literature exists, is it research based or purely speculative (untested)?
3. Is the literature tied together by any common conceptual or theoretical frameworks?
4. What do "state of the art" articles suggest about the adequacy of existing theoretical work on the topic? Are new perspectives, organization, or refinement needed?
5. What types of information or data do I have direct access to: clinical observations, field notes, computerized data files?
6. What unique resources do I as theory builder have access to that would facilitate my theory-building efforts: extensive library collection, computer facilities, clinical research projects with ready access to subjects?
7. What is my personal judgment about the approach to theory building that would be the most productive for me to pursue now on my topic of interest?

Carefully examine your answers to these questions. While more than one approach may be possible, the approach that is the most workable overall should get your first consideration. Should the first choice become unsatisfactory at a later date, then an alternative approach may be considered.

By *putting together* the decision about the *element* of theory and the *approach* most suited to the topic of interest, the choice of a specific *strategy* for theory building should be clear. For example, assume that "empathy" is a topic of interest that showed a need for further work at the concept level. Moreover, assume that analysis appeared best suited for dealing with the extensive literature on this concept (Forsyth, 1979; 1980). Concept analysis would then be a reasonable strategy for further theory building on "empathy."

INTERRELATEDNESS OF STRATEGIES

Successful theory development need not limit itself to only one approach or strategy. As a theory is being constructed, using one strategy may lead the theorist directly to a second strategy that further develops the new theory. We have proposed nine strategies here: concept, statement, and theory analysis; concept, statement, and theory synthesis; and concept, statement, and theory derivation. These nine are not all inclusive of the possible strategies available for use although they are inherent within most of them (Aldous, 1970; Burr, 1973; Hage, 1972; Zetterberg, 1965). They are our conception of the best strategies to use in nursing theory development in its present state.

Using these nine strategies will demonstrate quickly to the active theorist that no one strategy is going to supply all the needs for theory construction that may arise. The theorist will need to determine what the current status of the theory is before selecting a strategy to use. Once the strategy is selected, it should be used until it fails to yield additional information about the topic of interest. When the limits of one strategy are reached, it is time to turn to another strategy.

We believe that the process of theory building is iterative. That is, the theorist must continue to use and repeat strategies until the level of desired sophistication in the theory is reached. This iterative process has been called "retroduction" by Hanson (1958). He described the process as using both induction and deduction sequentially to arrive at an adequate theoretical formulation. In effect, Hanson proposes that first the theorist identify several propositions that are fairly specific and induce from them one more general proposition. The second phase of retroduction is to use the new proposition to deduce some new, more specific propositions. This process adds considerably to the body of theoretical knowledge. It is, in fact, the way theory develops in the "real world."

The nine strategies we have proposed here have not been classified as inductive or deductive. It seems to us that the only "pure" inductive strategies are the synthesis ones since they are clearly data based. The other strategies, analysis and derivation, may involve theorizing both inductively and deductively. We have preferred to deemphasize the notions of induction and deduction in the strategy chapters, however, in order to keep the strategies as clear and practical as possible. The idea of retroduction makes a great deal more sense to us given the state of the art and the nature of theory in nursing.

For a theorist, the problem is often how to continue once one has begun an attempt at theory construction. Perhaps using some examples here might demonstrate how the strategies can be used interdependently. Let us assume that a theorist reads an article that presents a new theory. A theory analysis helps the theorist understand that the concepts in the theory do not have careful operational definitions. The theorist decides to use concept analysis to develop better operational definitions. While using these two analysis strategies, the theorist begins to see possibilities for new relationships between some of the concepts. When he finally decides to formulate statements reflecting those relationships, the statement synthesis strategy is used.

A second example might be a doctoral student who, during her studies, begins developing a concept she hopes to use in her dissertation. The beginning interest in the concept occurred during the student's clinical practice. After several small field studies, the concept was synthesized. Later, when other concepts needed to be linked to the new one, a statement derivation strategy was used to provide an appropriate structure for the concepts. Finally, after the student graduated, a theory synthesis strategy was ultimately completed. Another theorist, reading the student's discussion of the theory, decided to use it in another discipline, and so theory derivation was used.

As you can see, the strategies stand alone and yet are interdependent. Each strategy provides the theorist with unique information, and yet all of them yield productive ideas for further theory development.

As you work with the various strategies, you will become more comfortable with their use. You may even modify some of them or develop new strategies for your theory construction repertoire. The hallmark of successful theorists is that they allow themselves the freedom to play with ideas or strategies until those ideas or strategies fit the needs of the theorist.

SUMMARY

In this chapter we have dealt with the elements, approaches, and strategies of theory building. The elements of a theory are concepts, statements, and theories. Analysis, synthesis, and derivation are the approaches to theory building. By combining the elements with the approaches, we have constructed a nine-cell matrix of theory-building strategies. Multiple strategies may often be employed before the theory development process is complete.

REFERENCES

Aldous J: Strategies for developing family theory. J Marriage Fam 32: 250–257, 1970.

Baltes PB, Reese HW, Nesselroade JR: Life-Span Developmental Psychology: Introduction to Research Methods. Monterey, Calif.: Brooks/Cole, 1977.

Bloom BS (ed.): Taxonomy of Educational Objectives. Handbook 1. Cognitive Domain. New York: McKay, 1956.

Brodbeck M: Models, meaning, and theories. In (M Brodbeck, ed.), Readings in the Philosophy of the Social Sciences. New York: Macmillan, 1968.

Burr JW: Theory Construction in Sociology of the Family. New York: Wiley, 1973.

Forsyth GL: Exploration of empathy in nurse-client interaction. Adv Nurs Sci 1(2): 53–61, 1979.

Forsyth GL: Analysis of the concept of empathy: Illustration of one approach. Adv Nurs Sci 2(2): 33–42, 1980.

Hage J: Techniques and Problems of Theory Construction in Sociology. New York: Wiley, 1972.

Hanson NR: Patterns of Discovery. Cambridge: Cambridge Univ. Press, 1958.

Hardy ME: Theories: Components, development, evaluation. Nurs Res 23: 100–107, 1974.

Hempel CG: Philosophy of Natural Science. Englewood Cliffs, N.J.: Prentice-Hall, 1966.

Maccia ES, Maccia GS: Development of Educational Theory Derived from Three Educational Theory Models. Columbus, Ohio: The Ohio State Univ. (Project No. 5-0638), 1966.

Reynolds P: A Primer in Theory Construction. Indianapolis: Bobbs-Merrill, 1971.

Riehl JP, Roy C: Theory and models. In (JP Riehl and C Roy, eds.), Conceptual Models for Nursing Practice. 2d ed. New York: Appleton-Century-Crofts, 1980.

Zetterberg HL: On Theory and Verification in Sociology. Totowa, N.J.: Bedminster Press, 1965.

ADDITIONAL READINGS

Readers who wish to do additional reading about theory and approaches to theory development may find the sources below of interest. (An asterisk indicates a reference for the advanced reader.)

*Blalock HM: Theory Construction: From Verbal to Mathematical Formulations. Englewood Cliffs, N. J.: Prentice-Hall, 1969.

*Brodbeck M: Models, meaning and theories. In (M Brodbeck, ed.), Readings in the Philosophy of the Social Sciences. New York: Macmillan, 1968, 579–600.

*Broudy H, Ennis R, Krimerman L (eds.): The Philosophy of Educational Research. New York: John Wiley, 1973.

Chinn PL (ed.): Advances in Nursing Theory Development. Rockville, Md.: Aspen, 1983.

Dubin R: Theory Building. 2d ed. New York: Free Press, 1978.

Fawcett J: A framework for analysis and evaluation of conceptual models of nursing. Nurse Ed 5: 10–14, 1980.

Fawcett J: The relationship between theory and research: A double helix. Adv Nurs Sci 1(1): 49–62, 1978.

Hardy ME: Perspectives on knowledge and role theory. In (ME Hardy & ME Conway, eds.), Role theory. New York: Appleton-Century-Crofts, 1978, 1–15.

Hempel CG: Philosophy of Natural Science. Englewood Cliffs, N. J.: Prentice-Hall, 1966.

Jacox A: Theory construction in nursing: An overview. Nurs Res 23: 4–13, 1974.

*Kuhn TS: The Structure of Scientific Revolutions. 2d ed. Chicago: Univ. of Chicago, 1970.
*Lakatos I, Musgrave A (eds.): Criticism and the Growth of Knowledge. Cambridge: Cambridge Univ., 1970.
Meleis AI: Theoretical Nursing: Development and Progress. Philadelphia: Lippincott, 1985.
Newman M: Theory Development in Nursing. Philadelphia: Davis, 1979.
Platt JR: Strong inference. Science 146: 347–352, 1964.
Rudner R: Philosophy of Social Science. Englewood Cliffs, N. J.: Prentice-Hall, 1966.
Wallace WL: The Logic of Science in Sociology. Chicago: Aldine-Atherton, 1971.

PART II
Concept Development

INTRODUCTION TO CONCEPT DEVELOPMENT

Concept development is a critical but often neglected approach to theory development in nursing and indeed in many scientific disciplines. The very basis of any theory depends on the identification and explication of the concepts to be considered in it. Yet many attempts to describe, explain, or predict phenomena start without a clear understanding of what is to be described, explained, or predicted. The next three chapters will focus on ways to develop concepts systematically.

Concept development is needed when one of three situations occurs. The first situation requiring concept development is one in which few concepts or no concepts are available in the theorist's focal area of interest. In this case the theorist must somehow obtain or invent concepts that are relevant to the phenomenon of concern. Either concept derivation (Chapter 5) or concept synthesis (Chapter 4) would be useful strategies to use.

The second situation requiring concept development is one in which concepts are already available in the area of interest but they are unclear, outmoded, or unhelpful. In this situation the theorist might choose to do a concept analysis (Chapter 3) of one or more of the unclear concepts in an effort to refine and clarify the concept. If the concepts are outmoded, then concept derivation (Chapter 5) might provide new ones that could provide useful insights.

The third situation requiring concept development is one in which a lot of theoretical literature or a lot of research on a topic of interest exists, but somehow the literature and the research do not match. This does not occur often. However, on occasion theorists may be working at one level on an area of interest and researchers or practitioners are working at another level and there is no clear bridge between the two. This has in fact happened in some of the nursing diagnosis work. When this occurs, careful concept development on some of the bridge concepts can be very helpful. The most useful strategy for this kind of work is often concept derivation (Chapter 5).

When you are trying to decide where to start with theory development, it might help to ask some questions before you begin. Such things as the level of theory development, the type of available literature, and the direction of the literature in the focal area of interest will all provide clues about where to begin. If any of the three situations above are predominant then one of the concept development strategies is the best place to begin.

Careful concept development is the basis of any attempt to describe or explain phenomena. It is also prerequisite to any adequate theory. By using one of the strategies discussed in the next three chapters, you will get off to a good start in your efforts at theory development.

3
Concept
Analysis

DEFINITION AND DESCRIPTION

Concept analysis is a strategy that allows us to examine the attributes or characteristics of a concept. Concepts contain within them the defining characteristics or attributes that permit us to decide which phenomena are good examples of the concept and which are not. Concepts are mental constructions; they are our attempts to order our environmental stimuli. Concepts, therefore, represent categories of information that contain defining attributes. Concept analysis is a formal, linguistic exercise to determine those defining attributes. The analysis itself must be rigorous and precise but the end product is always tentative. The reasons for this tentativeness stem from the fact that two people will often come up with somewhat different attributes for the same concept in their analyses and from the fact that scientific and general knowledge changes so quickly that what is "true" today is "not true" tomorrow.

Concept analysis encourages communication. If we are precise about carefully defining the attributes of the concepts we use in theory development and in research, we will make it far easier to promote understanding among our colleagues about the phenomena being discussed.

PURPOSE AND USES

The basic purpose of concept analysis is to distinguish between the defining attributes of a concept and its irrelevant attributes. It is a process of determining the likeness and unlikeness between concepts. By breaking a concept into its simpler elements, it is easier to determine its internal structure. Since we have already said in Chapter 2 that a concept is expressed by a word or a term in language (Reynolds, 1971), an analysis of a concept must, perforce, be an analysis of the descriptive word and its use. Concept analysis is ultimately only a careful examination and description of a word and its uses in the language coupled with an explanation of how it is "like" and "not like" other related words. We are concerned with both actual and possible uses of words that convey concept meanings.

Concept analysis is useful for several reasons. It can be useful in refining ambiguous concepts in a theory. It can help clarify those overused vague concepts that are prevalent in nursing practice so that everyone who subsequently uses the term will be speaking of the same thing. And concept analysis results in a precise operational definition that by its very nature has construct validity; that is, it will accurately reflect its theoretical base.

Concept analysis is an excellent way to begin examining information in preparation for research or theory construction. The results yield to the theorist or investigator a basic understanding of the underlying attributes of the concepts. This helps to clearly define the problem and to allow the investigator or theorist to construct hypotheses that accurately reflect the relationships between the concepts.

But perhaps the two most fruitful uses of concept analysis are in tool development and in developing nursing diagnoses. Nunnally (1978) has spoken to the need for careful conceptual development for research instruments. The results of concept analysis—the operational definition, list of defining attributes, and antecedents—can provide the scientist with an excellent beginning for a new tool or an excellent way to evaluate an old one. To begin a new tool, items could be constructed to reflect each of the defining attributes. Questions could be constructed to determine whether proposed antecedents occurred. With careful psychometric testing, the new tool could be useful for continuing research by interested scientists. The results of concept analysis are also useful in evaluating existing instruments. The instruments to be used in a research project could be examined in light of the results of the concept analysis to determine if the instruments accurately reflect the defining attributes of the relevant concepts.

The other primary use of concept analysis is in developing or evaluating nursing diagnoses. In many cases, nursing diagnoses have been developed consensually or in practice settings without thoroughly considering the theoretical or moral issues relating to assigning labels to clients or placing clients into diagnostic categories. It is not in the purview of this book to deal with the moral issues. However, it is within our purview to suggest that conducting a thorough concept analysis for any potential diagnosis would greatly facilitate taxonomic work and would thoroughly ground the nursing diagnosis in the pertinent theoretical and research literature. That is, each nursing diagnosis should be treated as a separate concept and should be analyzed independently. Most nursing diagnoses are written with three components—the health problem, the etiology, and the defining signs and symptoms (Gordon, 1982). These three components closely parallel the results of concept analysis—antecedents (etiology), defining characteristics (defining signs and symptoms), and operational definition (health problem). It seems reasonable to suggest using the two processes iteratively to improve our taxonomies and contribute to theory development simultaneously.

SPECIFIC PROCEDURES

According to Wilson (1969), the steps of concept analysis are:

1. Select a concept.
2. Determine the aims or purposes of analysis.
3. Identify all uses of the concept that you can discover.
4. Determine the defining attributes.
5. Construct a model case.
6. Construct borderline, related, contrary, invented, and illegitimate cases.
7. Identify antecedents and consequences.
8. Define empirical referents.

The steps in conducting a concept analysis will be discussed as if they were sequential. In fact, however, many of these steps occur simultaneously. Often some revision must be made in an earlier step because of information or ideas arising from a later one. This is to be expected. The iterative nature of the process results in a much cleaner, more precise analysis.

Select a Concept

The first step is often the hardest. Concept selection should be done with care. It is best to choose a concept in which you are already interested, one that is associated with your work, or one that has always "bothered" you.

It is important to avoid primitive terms that can only be defined by giving examples. It is equally important to avoid "umbrella" terms that are so broad they may encompass several meanings and confuse the analysis. Generally, concept selection should reflect the topic or area of greatest interest to you. Unexplored concepts can be found in nursing practice, can be generated from nursing research studies, or can be drawn from a theory that is as yet incomplete or that has concepts that are unclear.

Aims of Analysis

The second step in a concept analysis is to determine the *aims* or *purposes* of the analysis. This second step helps focus attention on exactly what use you intend to make of the results of your effort. It essentially answers the question, "Why am I doing this analysis?"

Some aims of an analysis might be to clarify the meaning of an existing concept, to develop an operational definition, or to add to existing theory. Another aim might be to distinguish between the normal, ordinary language usage of the concept and the scientific usage of the same concept. There are other possible purposes. The important thing is to decide for yourself, in advance, why you are interested in conducting a concept analysis. This definition of purpose is useful if as you begin to determine the defining attributes you discover several very dissimilar uses of the concept. The selection you make regarding which specific use of the concept you will choose should reflect the aims of the analysis.

Identify Uses of the Concept

The next step is to identify as many uses of the concept as you can find. To accomplish this, you may use dictionaries, thesauruses, colleagues, and available literature. At this initial stage *do not limit* yourself to only one aspect of the concept. You *must* consider *all* uses of the term. Ignoring the physical aspects of a concept and focusing only on the psychosocial, for instance, may deprive you of a great deal of valuable information. Remember to include both implicit as well as explicit uses of the concept. Extensive reading in as many different sources as possible is invaluable. This review of literature helps you support or validate your ultimate choices of the defining attributes.

For instance, if you were examining the concept of "coping" you would discover that not only are there psychological uses for the term but there are copings on buildings, coping saws, a method of trimming a falcon's beak called coping, and a coping that is an ecclesiastical garment similar to a cloak. All of these uses of the term must be included in your final analysis.

Occasionally, once you have identified *all* the usages of the concept, both ordinary and scientific, you may have to decide whether to continue to consider all aspects of the concept or only those pertinent to the scientific use. We generally feel that when possible you should continue to consider all aspects of the concept usage since that is likely to yield richer meanings. However, at times that will clearly be impractical or unhelpful. In these cases, use the aims of your analysis to guide your decision making.

As you collect the instances of concept use, you will find other instances that are similar or related to the concept being analyzed but are not quite the "real thing." Keep a list of these *related* and *borderline* instances. They will be helpful to you when you begin to construct borderline or related cases.

Determine Defining Attributes

When you have examined as many of the different instances of a concept as you can find, read through them all at once. As you read, make notes of the characteristics of the concept that appear over and over again. This list of characteristics, called defining or critical attributes, is often known as the list of *provisional criteria*. These criteria function very much like the criteria for making differential diagnoses in medicine. That is, they help you and others name the occurrence of a specific phenomenon as differentiated from another similar or related one.

Sometimes when you have gathered all the instances of a concept there will be a large number of possible meanings. A decision is clearly necessary regarding which will be the most useful and which will provide you the greatest help in relation to the *aims* of your analysis. You may decide to choose more than one meaning and continue analyzing using several meanings. For example, in the analysis of the concept of "attachment" at the end of this chapter we found that attachment can occur in both animate and inanimate forms. We chose to examine which attributes were common to both kinds and then to continue our analysis further to include the specific defining attributes for animate attachment since our area of interest was in mother-infant attachment (Avant, 1979). Consideration of the social or nursing care context in which the concept is to be used may be important in your decision as it was to us in the example. The final decision is up to you.

For instance, in our example of the concept "coping," the three characteristics that seemed to be most obvious among all those divergent uses of the term were (1) the attribute of covering something—an action, a cape, a window, a beak, (2) the attribute of protection—one's psyche, the garment under the cape, the flowers under the window, and (3) the attribute of adjusting or rebalancing. We decided that the idea of the coping saw was not relevant to the general concept since it does not reflect any of the three attributes that occur in all the other instances we have found. We will use this, in fact, as the example of an "illegitimate" case later in the analysis—one in which the term is used incorrectly in relation to its generally accepted meaning.

Develop Model Case(s)

At about the same time that you are developing the list of defining attributes, you should begin to develop a model case or cases. A model case is a "real life" example of the use of the concept that includes *all* the critical attributes and *no* attributes of any other concept. That is, the model case should be a pure case of the concept, a paradigmatic example. In fact, when a concept is reasonably new to you, a model case may come *first* in your analysis. At this stage it is often helpful and sometimes necessary to seek out a thoughtful colleague or two who can listen with a fresh ear as you talk through your examples. If there are flaws or errors you haven't seen, it is likely that someone else can spot them for you.

Basically, the model case is one that we are *absolutely sure* is an instance of the concept. Wilson (1969) suggests that the model case is one in which the analyst can say "Well, if *that* isn't an example of it, then nothing is."

In our coping example, for instance, the model case was stated as follows:

> A young woman is walking along a street wearing high heels and a silk dress. On her briefcase is a pouch with an umbrella in it. As she walks, it begins to rain heavily. She takes out her umbrella and raises it. She begins to run, but stumbles. She stops, removes her shoes quickly, and resumes running to the nearest shelter.

This model case includes all three of the critical attributes, covering, protection, and rebalancing. There are several other examples, or cases, of coping that could have been used instead. We tried to use one that was simple and commonplace for demonstration.

Construct Additional Cases

The next step is the construction of borderline, related, invented, and contrary cases. These cases are constructed for the purpose of providing examples of "not the concept" and for promoting further understanding of the concept being discussed.

Borderline cases are those examples or instances that contain some of the critical attributes of the concept being examined but not all of them. They may even contain most or all of the criteria but differ substantially in one of them, such as *length* of time or *intensity* of occurrence. These cases are inconsistent in some way and as such they help us see why the true or model case is not. In this way we help clarify our thinking about the defining or critical attributes of the true concept. Again using the coping example, a borderline case might be that of a college student who was facing a big exam. He had not studied until the evening before the test, when he "crammed all night." Halfway through the examination, he fell fast asleep and thereby flunked the test. This meets both attributes of covering and protection but breaks down when it comes to rebalancing.

Perhaps another example of a borderline case will make things even clearer. Since concepts act as a way of helping us classify things, we gave students an exercise in class. We asked them to categorize the contents of their closet. One student classified her clothes as "things I wear above my waist" and "things I wear below my waist." She was puzzled as to how to classify the belts since they were worn at the waist. This is a classic, indeed a concrete, example of a borderline case since the belt may fit into either category and yet really belongs to neither.

Related cases are instances of concepts that are related to the concept being studied but that do not contain the critical attributes. They are similar to the concept being studied. They are in some way connected to the main concept. The related cases help us understand how the concept being studied fits into the network of concepts surrounding it. Concepts that could be developed into related cases in our coping example, for instance, might be "stress," "conflict," "achievement," and "adaptation." Related cases are those cases that demonstrate ideas that are very similar to the main concept but that differ from them when examined closely.

Contrary cases are those that are clear examples of "not the concept." Again, Wilson (1969) suggests that it can be said of the contrary case, "Well, whatever the concept is, *that* is certainly not an instance of it." In our coping example, for instance, the contrary case might describe a young woman who is preparing dinner for a group of people. The roast burns on one end. She becomes hysterical, throws out the whole roast, and sends her guests home unfed. We can see from this example that whatever "coping" is, that young woman's behavior is not an example of it. It meets none of the three critical attributes we have said must pertain to an instance of coping—covering, protection, and rebalancing. Contrary cases are often very helpful to the analyst, since we often find it easier to say what something is not than what it is; and discovering what a concept is *not* helps us see in what ways the concept being analyzed is different from the contrary case. This, in turn, gives us information about what the concept should have as defining attributes if the ones from the contrary case are clearly excluded.

Invented cases are cases that are constructed using ideas outside our own experience. They often read like science fiction. Invented cases are useful when you are examining a very familiar concept such as "man," or "love," or one that is such a commonplace as to be taken for granted, such as "air." Often to get a true picture of the critical defining attributes, you must take the concept out of its ordinary context and put it into an invented one.

For example, suppose that a being from another planet visited earth. His physiology is such that when he becomes upset or frightened in our atmosphere, he floats straight up into the air, often bumping his head sharply on ceilings. He begins carrying a cement block in his backpack to keep him on the ground. In addition, he pads his helmet and wears it constantly. This is an example of coping in an invented case.

The last type of case is not always included in a concept analysis. It is the illegitimate case. These cases give an example of the concept term used improperly. In the case of the coping saw, the use of the term "coping" demonstrates neither the attribute of "covering" nor the one of "protection" and so is illegitimately used. These cases are helpful when you come across one meaning for a term that is completely different from all the others. It may have one or two of the critical attributes, but most of the attributes will not apply at all. In the "attachment" analysis at the end of this chapter, the term "attachment" as used to mean those pieces that fit onto a sewing machine contains only the attribute of "touch" and none of the other four.

Once the model cases are constructed, they must be compared to the critical or defining attributes one more time to ensure that all the critical attributes have been discovered. Sometimes, once the model case is constructed and compared with the other cases and the proposed critical attributes, some areas of overlap, vagueness, or contradiction will become apparent. It is at this point that further refinement becomes necessary. An analysis cannot be completed until there are no overlapping attributes and no contradictions between the defining attributes and the model case.

Identify Antecedents and Consequences

The next steps in a concept analysis are the identification of *antecedents* and *consequences*. Although these two steps are often ignored, they may shed considerable light on the social contexts in which the concept is generally used. They are also helpful in further refining the critical attributes. Something cannot be an antecedent and an attribute at the same time, for example. Antecedents are those events or incidents that must occur *prior to* the occurrence of the concept. For example, Ward (1986) gives a clear example of antecedents of role strain, identifying role conflict, role accumulation, rigidity of time and place, which role demands must be met, and the amount of activity prescribed by some roles as the antecedents. Consequences, on the other hand, are those events or incidents that occur as a *result* of the occurrence of the concept. For example, Rew (1986) indicates one consequence of intuition is discovery. In our coping example, one antecedent was an intensely stressful stimulus (the burned roast); the consequence was the regaining of balance. Another clear example presents itself to us: If we examine the concept of "pregnancy," one of the antecedents is clearly ovulation, while a consequence is some kind of delivery experience whether or not the pregnancy goes to term or produces a viable baby.

Antecedents and consequences are often extremely useful theoretically. Blalock (1969) has spoken of constructing theoretical models of determinants and results around a focal variable or construct. (See Chapter 10 for a more thorough discussion of his ideas.) His notion of determinants and results is very close to the notion of antecedents and consequences in concept analysis. Antecedents are also useful in helping the theorist identify underlying assumptions about the concept being studied. In our attachment example at the end of this chapter, you will see that one of the antecedents is the ability to distinguish between internal and external stimuli. This implies that an assumption of living, sentient beings has been made. Consequences are useful in determining often neglected ideas, variables, or relationships that may yield fruitful new research directions.

Define Empirical Referents

The final step is to determine the *empirical referents* for the critical attributes. In many cases the critical attributes and the empirical referents will be identical. However, there are times when the concept being analyzed is highly abstract and so are its critical attributes. In these cases, the question arises, "If we are to measure this concept or determine its existence in the real world, how do we do so?" Empirical referents are classes or categories of actual phenomena that by their existence or presence *demonstrate* the occurrence of the concept itself. As an example, "kissing" might be used as an empirical referent for the concept of "affection." In our "coping" example an empirical referent might be "ability to successfully solve a problem in a stressful situation."

Empirical referents, once identified, are extremely useful in instrument development because they are clearly linked to the theoretical base of the concept, thus contributing to both the content and construct validity of any new instrument. They are also very useful in practice since they provide the clinician with clear, observable phenomena by which to "diagnose" the existence of the concept in particular clients. The Boyd (1985), Rew (1986), Meize-Grochowski (1984), and Ward (1986) articles listed in the reference section of this chapter all have good examples of empirical referents.

ADVANTAGES AND LIMITATIONS

The main advantage of concept analysis is that it renders very precise theoretical as well as operational definitions for use in theory and research. Another advantage is that concept analysis could help clarify those terms in nursing that have become catch-phrases and hence have lost their meanings. A third advantage is its utility for tool development and nursing diagnosis. Additionally, the rigorousness of this intellectual exercise is extremely good practice in thinking.

The limitations are that the theorist must be painstaking and is likely to encounter pitfalls that will hinder the analysis.

Concept analysis clarifies the symbols used in communication. There are few firm rules for concept analysis. But there are some pitfalls you should avoid. These pitfalls tend to obscure the meanings you want to convey (Wilson, 1969). They are:

(1) The tendency to moralize when the concept being analyzed has some value implications. Many concepts hold some implicit if not explicit value to us. As we begin a concept analysis it is important to recognize that just choosing the concept demonstrates a bias on our part. We must be doubly careful, then, to treat the concept objectively as subject matter rather than subjectively as a persuasive weapon.

(2) The feeling of being absolutely in over your head. Since there are no firm rules in concept analysis, this may make you very anxious. There is no way we can say to you, "First do this, then do that, and when you have done so, all will be wonderful." We have attempted to give you guidelines, but the actual intellectual work must be yours. Once you have begun, the anxiety subsides and the fun begins.

(3) The feeling that concept analysis is too easy. Some people initially grow impatient with the process and tend to throw up their hands with the comment, "Well, everybody knows that term means so-and-so. Why do we need to keep on with this?" The point is that *not* everybody knows what it means. Concept analysis is not easy; it

is a vigorous intellectual exercise, but it is fruitful and useful and even enjoyable.

(4) The compulsion to analyze everything, or the "how-do-you-turn-it-off syndrome" as one of our students calls it. This occurs fairly often in students. The process of analysis somehow gets their creative juices flowing and they get very excited. The result is often that they don't want to stop. There are some concepts more worthy of analysis than others, but all analyses must finally come to an end. In addition, analysis is only one strategy in theory development. Some energy should be saved for the rest!

(5) The need to protect oneself from others' criticism or debate during the process of analysis. Good concept analysis cannot occur in a vacuum. Only the insights and criticisms of others can fully expand the analyst's ideas. The willingness to look foolish is one of the criteria for creativity. If you restrain yourself in discussions or fail to seek criticism because you may look "silly" or "dumb," you are cutting yourself off from successful concept development. In dealing with concept analysis, it is vital to say *something* and then trust that it will lead somewhere.

(6) The feeling that verbal facility equals thinking. There is sometimes a tendency to engage in superficial fluency instead of productive dialogue. The ability to explore all the avenues of investigation is important but time consuming. The results of hasty analysis are meager and unproductive. The idea is to reach a happy compromise between the two approaches.

(7) Another pitfall in concept analysis may occur if theorists attempt to add additional critical attributes because they see that their list is short. Doing so can confound the results of the analysis since many of the added attributes are not critical to the concept and may even overlap the antecedents and consequences. A rule of thumb is to "quit when you're done" with the original analysis.

Any or all of these pitfalls hinder analysis. A sense of proportion, a little risk taking, a sense of humor, and a low anxiety level are all helpful in the process of analysis. This is a new way of thinking for many people and as such requires a little getting used to in the beginning. It is a very important aspect to theory construction. Since concepts are the bricks of theory development, it is critical that they be structurally sound. If a theory contains careful concept analyses, all who read the theory or use it in practice will be able to clearly understand what is meant by the concepts within it and their relationships to each other.

Finally, concepts, even well-analyzed ones, can contribute only the basics of theory. Only when concepts are studied for relationships among them and relational statements constructed can real forward progress be made in theory construction.

UTILIZING THE RESULTS OF CONCEPT ANALYSIS

We have discussed several uses of the results of concept analysis. These are refining ambiguous terms in theory, education, research, and practice; providing operational definitions with a clear theoretical base; providing an understanding of the underlying attributes of a concept; facilitating instrument development in research; and providing assistance in the development of nursing diagnoses. However, once a concept has been analyzed, what is the next step for the theorist? This depends in part on the aims of the analysis. If one of the aims, for instance, was to develop an instrument, then the next step would be to construct items that would reflect the defining attributes of the concept. If the aim was to propose a nursing diagnosis, the next step would be to clinically validate the defining attributes. Using the empirical referents for the defining attributes and assessing clients for the presence or absence of the attributes would help substantiate the potential diagnosis. If the aim was to construct an operational definition, the next step would be to attempt to find a research instrument that accurately reflects the defining attributes of the concept.

It is clear that concept analysis alone will not provide useful theories for nursing education, research, or practice. It will only be when the concepts are linked to each other that useful theories will result. In the meantime, scientists, educators, and clinicians should continue to examine concepts critically in an effort to refine our knowledge and to discover what those linkages are.

SUMMARY

This chapter has described the process of concept analysis. This strategy employs the processes of analysis to extract the defining, or critical, attributes of a concept. There are no rules for accomplishing the analysis. Selection of the concept and the theorist's familiarity with the literature will have some impact on where the theorist begins. The steps in concept analysis include selecting the concept, determining the aims of analysis, identifying all uses of the concept, determining the defining or critical attributes of the concept, constructing model cases, constructing additional cases, defining identi-

fying antecedents and consequences, and defining empirical referents.

Concept analysis increases the richness of our vocabulary and
provides precise and rigorously constructed theoretical and operational definitions for use in theory and research. It is limited by the
level of theory that can be attained using only concepts. In the next
chapter we shall discuss another strategy, concept synthesis, which is
useful when there are no concepts to be analyzed about some specific
topic of interest.

PRACTICE EXERCISE AND ONE
ADDITIONAL EXAMPLE

To aid you with the subsequent practice exercise, we have presented
below a brief summary of a concept analysis of "attachment." This is
by no means a complete, formal analysis. It is presented merely to
show you how one looks as it is developed.

Concept: Attachment.
Aim of Analysis: Develop operational definition of theoretical concept.
Critical Attributes:
All cases of attachment:

1. Visual contact must have been made between the person and the
   object of attachment.
2. The object of attachment must have been touched by the person at
   some time during the process of attachment.
3. There must be some positive affect associated with the object of
   attachment.

Cases of animate attachment have in addition to the above:

4. There must be reciprocal interaction between the two parties in
   attachment.
5. Vocalization by at least one of the two parties is supportive of
   attachment process.

Model Cases
Person-to-Object Attachment

> A woman explains to her friend that she simply can't throw out
> her old bathrobe because she has had it since she married and is
> just too "attached to it."

Person-to-Person Attachment

An eight-month-old boy is playing in the room where his mother is sewing. As he plays, he occasionally looks around at her, or comes over and touches her. When she leaves the room, he cries and begins to search for her. When she returns, he climbs into her lap. She hugs him close and talks to him until he is ready to continue playing.

Contrary Case

A 22-year-old woman delivers a baby under general anesthesia and cesarean section as a result of abruptio placenta. The infant is about 26 weeks gestation and weighs 2 lbs. He is immediately transferred to the regional perinatal center 200 miles away. When the mother wakes from anesthesia, she is told she has a 2-lb. baby boy and also about his transfer. She is told the baby will stay in hospital until he weighs about 5 lbs. Due to postpartum complications, the mother is not released from the hospital for three weeks. Even though her husband brings reports of the baby, she says "Do I really have a baby?"

Borderline Case

Jeffrey is being seen at the health clinic for possible child abuse. Jeffrey is blind due to retrolental fibroplasia. He also has spastic cerebral palsy. Jeffrey's mother says she gets angry because he won't look at her or cuddle when she picks him up. When he cries too long, she hits him. This is borderline attachment because two defining characteristics, touch and vocalization, are met. Visual contact, positive affect, and reciprocal interaction are absent or severely diminished. Attachment may still occur, but it will be difficult.

Related Cases

Love	Deprivation
Separation	Dependency
Detachment	Symbiosis

Illegitimate Case

A salesman demonstrating a new sewing machine makes a point of explaining "the most useful attachment—the buttonholer."

Antecedents

1. Ability to distinguish between internal and external stimuli.
2. Ability to receive and respond to cues of the persons involved in attachment process.

Consequences

1. Proximity-maintaining behavior
2. Separation anxiety

Empirical Referents. Examples

1. Eye-to-eye contact
2. Patting, stroking, holding hands, etc.
3. Speaking positively about the person
4. Speaking, singing, reading to the person

Practice Exercise

Analyze the concept of "play" using the foregoing analysis as a guide.

Some of your critical attributes probably were similar to the ones below:

1. Movement or activity
2. One animate entity
3. Voluntariness or choice
4. Expectation of diversion or pleasure
5. Novelty or unpredictability
6. Creativity

Did you remember to include the ideas "play on words," "play in the steering wheel," "play" as in a drama, and so forth?

Using the critical attributes above, develop a model case that includes all of them.

What are some related concepts? How about "games," "work," "exercise," "performance," "imitate," "sport"?

Try developing a contrary case using "work" as "not play." Use the concept "exercise" as a borderline case.

Complete the analysis using the outline given.

REFERENCES

Avant K: Nursing diagnosis: Maternal attachment. Adv Nurs Sci 2(1): 45–56, 1979.
Blalock HM: Theory Construction from Verbal to Mathematical Formulations. Englewood Cliffs, N. J.: Prentice-Hall, 1969.
Boyd C: Toward an understanding of mother-daughter identification using concept analysis. Adv Nurs Sci 7(3): 78–86, 1985.
Gordon M: Nursing Diagnosis: Process and Application. New York: McGraw-Hill, 1982.
Meize-Grochowski R: An analysis of the concept of trust. J Adv Nurs 9: 563–572, 1984.

Nunnally J: Psychometric Theory. New York: McGraw-Hill, 1978.

Rew L: Intuition: Concept analysis of a group phenomenon. Adv Nurs Sci 8 (2): 21–28, 1986.

Reynolds PD: A Primer in Theory Construction. Indianapolis: Bobbs-Merrill, 1971.

Ward C: The meaning of role strain. Adv Nurs Sci 8(2): 39–49, 1986.

Wilson J: Thinking with Concepts. New York: Cambridge Univ. Press, 1969.

ADDITIONAL READINGS

Arakelian M: An assessment and nursing application of the concept of locus of control. Adv Nurs Sci 3(1): 25–42, 1980.

Carnevali D: Conceptualizing, a nursing skill. In (PH Mitchell, ed.), Concepts Basic to Nursing. 2d ed. New York: McGraw-Hill, 1977.

Carper B: Fundamental patterns of knowing in nursing. Adv Nurs Sci 1(1): 13–23, 1978.

Chinn PL, Jacobs K: A model for theory development in nursing. Adv Nurs Sci 1(1): 1–12, 1978.

Englemann S: Conceptual Learning. San Rafael, Calif.: Dimensions, 1969.

Hempel CG: Fundamentals of Concept Formation in Empirical Science. Chicago: Univ. of Chicago Press, 1952.

Klausmeier HJ, Ripple RE: Learning and Human Abilities. Chapter 11. New York: Harper & Row, 1971.

Matthews C, Gaul A: Nursing diagnosis from the perspective of concept attainment and critical thinking. Adv Nurs Sci 2(1): 17–26, 1979.

Norris CM: Restlessness: A nursing phenomenon in search of meaning. Nurs Outlook 23: 103–107, 1975.

Popper KR: Conjectures and Refutations. 4th ed. London: Rutledge & Kegan Paul, 1972.

Rawnsley M: The concept of privacy. Adv Nurs Sci 2(2): 25–32, 1980.

Smith J: The idea of health: A philosophical inquiry. Adv Nurs Sci 3(3): 43–50, 1981.

Stern PN: Grounded theory methodology: Its uses and processes. Image 12 (2): 20–23, 1980.

4

Concept
Synthesis

DEFINITION AND DESCRIPTION

Concept synthesis is a strategy for developing concepts based on observation or other forms of empirical evidence. As in all synthesis strategies, concept synthesis is based on observation or evidence. The data may come from direct observation, quantitative evidence, or literature. The process of concept synthesis is one of the most exciting ways of beginning theory building. It permits the theorist to use clinical experience as one place to begin.

Concepts are ordered information about the attributes of one or more things that enables us to differentiate them from other thing(s) (Wilson, 1969). The theorist using this strategy must invent a new way of grouping, or ordering, information about some event or phenomenon, when the relevant dimensions one should use to do so are unclear or unknown: In a very real sense, one must start from scratch.

Concept synthesis as a creative behavior is not something requiring genius. New concepts often develop from very ordinary activities. In fact, all of us who think form new concepts, or categories, as our experiences in the world increase. When children begin to learn, they begin to place things into categories. These are not always *logical* categories at first, but they become so as the child learns to associate things that are similar in some way. As the child's experience increases, he or she begins to compare new information with the already learned concepts, or categories, of things. If the new information fits one of the previously existing concepts, or categories, it is easily assimilated. If the new information does not fit any previously existing concept or category then the child must develop a strategy for dealing with the new information. He or she has one of three choices: (1) mislabel the information by putting it in an old category, (2) deny the new information altogether, or (3) develop a new concept (Hunt, 1962; Stevenson, 1972; Spitzer, 1977).

Often help in this effort is available from the child's environment, from a parent or teacher for instance. If a child has always categorized animals with four legs and a tail as "doggie" and then comes up against an animal with four legs and a tail but it has an udder and goes "moo" and is four feet tall, there will be some discrepancy in this instance between the new animal and a "doggie." The parent may help the child solve the problem by saying "That is a cow." We, as adults, are not always so lucky. When we encounter a new phenomenon in our own experience, there is not always someone around to tell us what the new concept is. We must then invent our own label to explain the new phenomenon. This, in effect, is concept formation, the precursor of concept synthesis.

Concept synthesis can occur in any one of several ways: (1) by discovering new dimensions of "old" concepts; (2) by examining sets of related concepts for similarities or discrepancies; or (3) by observing new phenomena or clusters of phenomena that have not been described previously. When the discovery of a new concept has been made, a label is invented for the concept that will demonstrate the meaning and allow for communication about it. This concept should include its defining attributes so that the reader can determine what is and what is not the new concept.

PURPOSE AND USES

The purpose of concept synthesis is to generate new ideas. It provides a method of examining data for new insights that can add to theoretical development. New concepts add richness to our vocabulary and point to new areas for study.

Concept synthesis is also useful for what Dray (1959) has described as "explanatory generalizations." He speaks of these occurring in a process of synthesis that ". . . allows us to refer to x, y, and z collectively as 'a so and so.' " It is, in effect, explaining by finding an appropriate classification for the phenomenon under concern and naming it. Gordon (1982) has called this same process "pattern recognition." This is a particularly useful strategy for developing nursing diagnoses. In fact, almost any new diagnosis, new syndrome, or new taxonomy represents an attempt at concept synthesis. Whenever a new phenomenon or cluster of phenomena are described empirically or generated from data, the process of concept synthesis has already begun.

Concept synthesis is useful in several areas: (1) in areas where there is little or no concept development, (2) in areas where concept development is present but has had no real impact on theory or practice, and (3) in areas where observations of phenomena are available but not yet classified or named.

SPECIFIC PROCEDURES

There are three approaches to concept synthesis: qualitative, quantitative, and literary. A qualitative approach requires using sensory data such as that gained from listening or observing to obtain information. It speaks to properties of things without assigning a numerical value to the amount of the property present. As the data are collected, they are examined for similarities and differences much as one would in using a grounded theory approach (Glaser & Strauss, 1967). Basically, qualitative synthesis involves recognizing patterns among observations. Harris's (1986) study of cultural values and decisions regarding circumcision is a good example of qualitative synthesis. Using a grounded approach, Harris interviewed parents, nurses, and physicians about newborn males. These categories were discovered: circumcision reasoning, cultural decision making, and cultural franchising. These three main concepts were then placed within an explanatory model of cultural decision making about circumcision.

A quantitative approach requires the use of numerical data. You may use any studies—experimental or nonexperimental single case or group designs—as long as they provide quantitative data about the phenomenon of interest. Statistical methods may be employed to extract clusters of attributes comprising a new concept as well as depicting those attributes that do not belong to the concept. Measures such as Q sorts, factor analysis, and Delphi techniques are especially helpful for generating meaningful clusters. Oldaker's study (1986) of normal adolescents' psychologic symptomatology is a good example of a quantitative concept synthesis. From several indices of psychological symptoms and personality, Oldaker used principal axis factor analysis to synthesize four concepts related to identity confusion: intimacy, negative identity, diffusion of time perspective, and diffusion of industry.

A literary approach involves the careful examination of literature for the purpose of acquiring new insights about phenomena of interest. This examination may yield previously unrecognized concepts for study. Particular to literary concept synthesis is the idea that the literature *itself* becomes the data base. Rogge's (1985) historical study of nursing activities in the Civil War is a good example. Using literature only, she generated a set of 11 categories of nursing interventions: information gathering, expressive, informative, injunctive, purveyor, receptive, corporeal, socializing, tacit, tactile, and transcendental. These interventions were then classified into four dimensions of practice that she labeled preparatory, inceptive, recuperative, and thanatological.

There are several steps in concept synthesis. We will discuss them sequentially but, as in most of the strategies, they are really iterative. That is, one does not progress from step to step but may cycle through steps several times or go back and forth between steps. One study refers to this process as becoming "theoretically saturated" (Glaser & Strauss, 1967). To do this one must become thoroughly familiar with the area of interest by using many resources including literature reviews and case studies. All provide potential sources of data.

As you become saturated, begin to classify the data you have acquired. The system of classification need not be rigorous. Indeed, it is better if the system stays fairly loose at this stage. While you are classifying the data, look for clusters of phenomena that seem to relate closely to each other or that overlap considerably and combine them. To do this clustering requires only that each classification category be compared to each other category. This can be done using factor analysis on a computer but is not really difficult when done by the theorist using visual inspection.

Once the clusters have been discovered and combined where possible, examine them for any hierarchical structure. If there are clusters that appear very similar but one is of a broader nature than the other, it may be helpful to reduce the two clusters into one higher-order concept. When the new concept has been reduced as much as possible, a label should be chosen for it that accurately describes it and that facilitates communication about it.

The next step in concept synthesis is to verify the new concept empirically and modify it if necessary. Verification involves a return to literature, field studies, data collection, and colleagues to discover if the concept is empirically supported. That is, do any of these data sources provide additional information that will expand, clarify, negate, or limit the concept? This process continues until the theorist is satisfied that no new information is being received. At this point the process stops and the new concept is considered adequate. The new concept should then be described in a theoretical definition that includes its defining attributes.

The final step in concept synthesis is to determine, if possible, where the new concept fits into existing theory in the area. Consideration should be given to the new insights and new approaches to research and practice the new concept makes possible. There may even be times when a concept is so radically different from current theoretical positions that a whole new field of study emerges, much as the discovery of microbes generated the field of bacteriology, or an existing system of thinking is completely changed, as when the concept of relativity completely changed the orientation of the field of physics.

Perhaps some examples of concept synthesis will make the steps easier to comprehend.

We will use a qualitative example first. Let us suppose that you are interested in gerontology. As you begin to examine case records and talk to aging persons you see that many of them talk of loneliness, isolation, being alone, "not getting around" like they used to, and friends dying. You decide to make two classifications of data called "limited mobility" and "loneliness." You put all the different instances that you observe of these behaviors under the appropriate category.

Once you have seen many elderly people, you can begin to form clusters of data that seem to overlap each other. When you look at the data categories of "limited mobility" and "loneliness" you find that almost all the behaviors are the same. Since this is the case, you can combine the two categories into one category, "loneliness." However, as you continue to examine your data, you find that a third category, "reduced social support," also overlaps the category of "loneliness" but is somewhat broader in scope. Since this broader scope may be desirable in beginning concept development, you decide to reduce the categories of "loneliness" and "reduced social support" to a higher-order concept. To do this requires that you choose a label for the new concept that better reflects its scope. You choose the label "social isolation," which implies not only being alone or isolated but also the idea of reduced social contact (Hurley, 1986).

The next two steps would then be to verify the new concept of social isolation empirically to clarify its meaning and boundaries and then to fit it into existing theories. If the concept is considered valid, it might lend new insights into the study of clinical depression in the elderly by helping to distinguish between personality disorders and situational crises.

Our second example will be an actual quantitative study that resulted in concept synthesis. Psychologists Kobasa et al. (1979) were studying the effects of life stress on middle- and upper-eschelon managers. What they discovered surprised them—of the managers who were identified by high-stress levels as at risk for illness, about one-third had not had any or at least few illnesses. What made these executives different? Everything they knew about stress suggested that they should be sick. Was it something in these executives' responses to stressful events that protected them from illness? As a result of these questions, Kobasa et al. set up several studies to collect data on the categories of "openness to change," "involvement," and "control over events." As the data were analyzed the categories were reduced slightly to become "challenge," "commitment," and "control." Finally, the concept label "hardiness" was used to accurately reflect the three combined categories. Additional studies have since validated the concept for some occupations but not entirely for others. The studies continue. However, the new concept has already made a major impact on stress theory (Kobasa, 1979a; 1979b; Kobasa et al., 1979).

Our final example demonstrates the use of qualitative and quantitative concept synthesis combined. Clunn (1984) used grounded theory combined with questionnaires to study the cues nurses used to formulate a nursing diagnosis of potential for violence and whether the nurses discriminated between degrees of violent behavior. Using interviews, literature, and scales, 11 concepts were synthesized from Clunn's study: medical history, content of verbalizations, peer relationships, social history, background factors, purposeful motor actions, nonpurposeful motor actions, intensity or emotionality of verbalizations, pervasive affective state, labile emotional reactions, and cognitive indicators of disequilibrium. From these 11 concepts, Clunn synthesized three majors factors, interaction, action, and awareness, as the three cue categories most used in diagnosing potential for violence. These three factors emerged in both the qualitative and the quantitative portions of the study. Her findings indicated that the actual cues and categories of cues nurses used in assessing the client's potential for violence were similar but the patterns that were salient for some groups of nurses (e.g., emergency room) were not the same as those for other groups (e.g., state hospital).

Several factors will make concept synthesis easier to practice. The first factor is a good memory. It is very important to be thoroughly familiar with one's own field of interest. It is equally important to be able to retain a significant amount of that knowledge in your memory. In this way, phenomena that "don't compute" with existing ways of thinking become more obvious.

Because memory is fallible, it is very useful for theorists to develop a notebook of memos to themselves. In this notebook, observations should be carefully recorded. These may be directly observed phenomena, statistical findings, or information summaries from literature. Both at the time of writing the memo and at the time the theorist reviews the notebook, insights and interpretations of the data should be added to the memo. These interpretive notes form the basis for developing classifications in both initial concept synthesis efforts and in efforts to develop higher concepts at a later time (Schatzman & Strauss, 1973).

Another factor that facilitates concept synthesis is the ability to observe. Obviously, a keen observer is more likely to see new phenomena than one who never looks. This skill is not inborn. It is acquired with practice. If you feel you are not a careful observer, try Practice Exercise 1 at the end of this chapter.

A corollary to the skill of observation is the skill of evaluating evidence. This ability to look at data, determine its value, and extract the new ideas can be learned also. The reader is referred to the additional readings on evaluating research at the end of this chapter that may help you in evaluating evidence.

The last factor that influences concept synthesis is openness to new ideas. This implies, at least, a freedom from the fear of discovering something new. Many nurses practice nursing precisely as they were taught and have little inclination to question or experiment with new ways of doing or thinking about things. Change to many people is very threatening and certainly synthesizing a new concept will initiate some change, if only in thinking. Therefore, before concept synthesis can occur, the nurse must be willing to allow the possibility of new ideas.

New ideas come to us from all our senses. Most of us are verbally and mathematically trained but have no practice relying on taste, smell, or vision or touch to help us arrive at new ideas. It is often helpful to think divergently by forcing ourselves to use other than our verbal or mathematics skills to get new ideas about phenomena.

Coupled with the idea of using all our senses to help us generate new concepts is the admonition to take plenty of time. The process of synthesis is like creating something; it cannot be accomplished quickly. Ideas take time to develop or "incubate." Relax and don't push yourself.

ADVANTAGES AND DISADVANTAGES

The advantage of using concept synthesis as a strategy is that it provides a mechanism for creating something new from data already available. It provides new insights and adds texture and richness to the fabric of developing theory. It is especially useful in generating potential nursing diagnoses.

The disadvantages are that concept synthesis takes time and requires the theorist to be open to risk taking. The theorist must begin with raw data and attempt to conceive a new idea from it. Sometimes, but not often, this happens quickly. More often, it happens only after considerable time and thought.

Then, the step of verifying concepts also takes time. This is when the theorist feels most uncomfortable. What if the new concept can't be verified? The fear of being wrong is a powerful one, especially when the theorist may view the new concept as a "brain child" and is very attached to it. The necessity here is for the theorist to remain objective and scientific. If the concept is truly data based, it should come through the verification with only minor revisions.

Finally, concepts in themselves are only useful to describe a phenomenon. They do not provide for prediction or control. It is only when concepts are related to each other in statements that we have the possibility of a theory.

UTILIZING THE RESULTS OF CONCEPT SYNTHESIS

We have said that concept synthesis is useful when there is a need for new concepts or new uses for old ones or when we need to explain something by classifying it. But what do you do with a new concept once you've synthesized it?

Several things can and should be done. The first of these is to verify the concept or validate its existence. This is very much like establishing content validity in research, and the same methods can be used for either task. Once it is validated, a good theoretical definition containing the defining attributes should be written. Once this is accomplished, the new concept should be shared by publishing it.

Valid new concepts are useful in science and in practice. In education, the new concept could be used to describe nursing phenomena to students in a meaningful way or to classify patient needs or nursing actions. In practice the new concept may give clinicians new insights into patient problems, new nursing diagnoses, and possible new nursing interventions. In research and theory building, the new concept may provide fruitful new hypotheses or induce a change in thinking about some phenomenon of concern that in turn will generate more research. Any of these activities result in knowledge development in the discipline.

SUMMARY

In this chapter the strategy of concept synthesis has been explained. This strategy employs pulling together various elements of data into a pattern or relationship not clearly seen before so as to form a new whole or new concept. The steps of concept synthesis include becoming thoroughly familiar with an area of interest, loosely classifying the data you have acquired about the area of interest, looking for and combining clusters of classified phenomena that seem to relate closely or overlap each other, choosing a label for the cluster that accurately represents the phenomenon and that will facilitate communication about it, verifying the new concept empirically, and determining if or where the new concept fits into current theory and practice.

Concept synthesis is a highly creative activity and may add significant new information to a given area of interest. The strategy is limited by the length of time needed for full concept development and by the fact that concepts alone do not provide predictive potential.

PRACTICE EXERCISES

Exercise 1. Observing
Choose an object in your environment, such as a piece of equipment you use frequently or an object you handle every day. Spend ten minutes observing the object. Make a list of everything you see about it. How long was your list? If you saw only a few things go back and spend ten more minutes observing it. Is your list longer? Did you take the object apart and describe each piece separately? If not, why not? Now, go back and look again. Spend ten minutes listing all possible uses of the item. How long was the list? Did you describe uses for each *part* of the item as well as for the whole? If not, why not? Learning to be a keen observer requires that our stereotypes can be disposed of and that we keep an open and playful mind when we really *look* at something familiar.

Exercise 2. Memory
Without looking at one, draw a nondigital telephone dial. Put in the letters and numbers where they belong (Adams, 1979).

Very few people can do this right the first time. The exercise demonstrates how we may *think* we have all the data we need, because we use the phone every day after all, but are *so* familiar with the object we no longer really *see* it. Try this exercise again with an object you use every day at work. First, draw it without looking, then go back and draw it again while you look at it. How did the two differ?

Exercise 3. Concept Synthesis
In order to facilitate your practice of the steps in concept synthesis, we have structured this exercise more than will be the case in reality. In fact, what we have done here is to present a kind of matrix used in morphological analysis to help get you started (Adams, 1979).

Let us assume that you and your staff are frustrated at the inefficient ways patients are transported from place to place in your hospital. You decide to discover a new concept of patient transportation. To construct the matrix you need at least three parameters. Let us assume you choose (1) the power source to be used, (2) the devices into which the patient will be put, and (3) the medium in or on which the device will move. Figure 4.1 is the matrix we constructed. Feel free to add additional columns if you want to do so.

Now pick one item at random from each of the three axes and

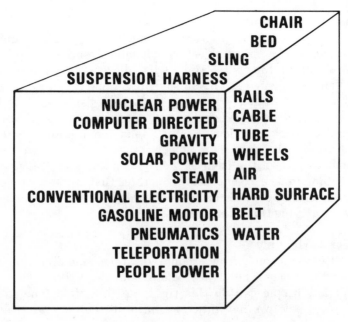

Figure 4.1. Three-Way Matrix

combine them. If, for instance, you got a bed with wheels that ran on people power, you have the conventional stretcher—not too helpful. But what if you got a bed on a track that was run by a computer? That *is* a new idea. Now try it several times. List the combinations. Now choose the two most likely new ideas. Choose a label that describes the new phenomenon. Let your imagination work here. If you got a combination of sling, pneumatic power, and tube, for instance, what could you call it? How about Pneuma-port? or Pneuma-sling? Sling-a-Pat? There are many possibilities.

The next two steps are to verify the concept empirically. In this exercise, verification would need to include exploration of whether or not the technology and the administrative and economic support were available to construct a prototype model. Once the model was constructed, pilot testing would demonstrate its feasibility, efficiency, and effectiveness. The last step is to determine if the prototype fits into existing systems of hospital care or if it requires a whole new system.

This brief exercise may seem very artificial, and it is; but it is one example of concept synthesis and should demonstrate the basic steps for you. Remember, practice makes perfect!

REFERENCES

Adams JL: Conceptual Blockbusting: A Guide to Better Ideas. 2d ed. New York: W. W. Norton, 1979.

Clunn P: Nurses' assessment of a person's potential for violence: Use of grounded theory in developing a nursing diagnosis. In (MJ Kim, GR Mc-Farland, & AM McLane, eds.), Classification of Nursing Diagnoses: Proceedings of the Fifth National Conference. St. Louis: Mosby, 1984, 376–393.

Dray W: "Explaining what" in history. In (P Gardiner, ed.), Theories of History. New York: The Free Press, 1959.

Glaser BG, Strauss AL: The Discovery of Grounded Theory: Strategies for Qualitative Research. Chicago: Aldine, 1967.

Gordon M: Nursing Diagnosis: Process and Application. New York: McGraw-Hill, 1982

Harris CC: Cultural values and the decision to circumcise. Image 18(3): 98–104, 1986.

Hunt EB: Concept Learning. New York: Wiley, 1962.

Hurley ME: Classification of Nursing Diagnoses: Proceedings of the Sixth National Conference. St. Louis: Mosby, 1986, 542.

Kobasa SC: Personality and resistance to illness. Amer J Commun Psychol 7: 413–423, 1979a.

Kobasa SC: Stressful life events, personality, and health: An inquiry into hardiness. J Pers Social Psychol 37: 1–11, 1979b.

Kobasa SC, Hiker RRJ, Maddi SR: Who stays healthy under stress? J Occupat Med 21: 595–598, 1979.

Oldaker S: Nursing diagnoses among adolescents. In (ME Hurley, ed.), Classification of Nursing Diagnoses: Proceedings of the Sixth National Conference. St. Louis: Mosby, 1986, 311–318.

Rogge MM: Development of a Taxonomy of Nursing Interventions: An Analysis of Nursing Care in the American Civil War. Unpublished doctoral dissertation. The Univ. of Texas at Austin, April, 1985.

Schatzman L, Strauss AL: Field Research. Englewood Cliffs, N. J.: Prentice-Hall, 1973.

Spitzer DR: Concept Formation and Learning in Early Childhood. Columbus, Ohio: Charles E. Merrill, 1977

Stevenson HW: Concept learning. In (HW Stevenson, ed.), Children's Learning. New York: Appleton-Century-Crofts, 1972, 308–322.

Wilson J: Thinking with Concepts. New York: Cambridge Univ. Press, 1969.

ADDITIONAL READINGS

Davitz JR, Davitz LL: A Guide: Evaluating Research Proposals in the Behavior Sciences. 2d ed. New York: Teachers College Press, 1977.

Kerlinger FN: Foundations of Behavioral Research. 2d ed. New York: Holt, Rinehart & Winston, 1973.

Klausmeier H: The nature of uses of concepts. In Learning and Human Abilities: Educational Psychology. 4th ed. New York: Harper & Row, 1975, 268–298.

Kleinmuntz B (ed.): Concepts and the Structure of Memory. New York: John Wiley & Sons, 1967.

Locke LF, Spirduso, WW: Proposals That Work: A Guide For Planning Research. New York: Teachers College Press, 1976.

Pines M: Psychological hardiness: The role of challenge in health. Psychol Today 14(7): 34–42, 98, 1980.

5
Concept
Derivation

DEFINITION AND DESCRIPTION

An analogy between phenomena in two fields is the basis for concept derivation. By looking at a new field of interest as an analog to a defined "parent" field, concepts for describing the new field may be derived. Further, by redefining concepts from the parent field to fit the new field, a new set of concepts is created. Thus, the newly defined concepts no longer rely on the parent field for meaning.

Concept derivation is applicable where a meaningful analogy can be made between one field that is conceptually defined and another that is not. Expressed more precisely, concept derivation consists of moving a concept (C_1) from one field of interest (F_1) to another field (F_2). In the process of transposing a concept, it is necessary that the concept (C_1) be redefined as a new concept (C_2) that fits the new field of study (F_2). This process is diagrammed in Figure 5.1. Thus C_1 leads to C_2, but F_1 and F_2 are *not* the same. Redefinition of C_1 results in a concept (C_2) that is based on but different from C_1.

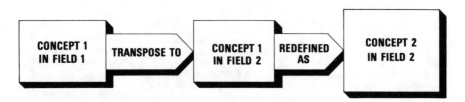

| CONCEPT 1 IN FIELD 1 | TRANSPOSE TO | CONCEPT 1 IN FIELD 2 | REDEFINED AS | CONCEPT 2 IN FIELD 2 |

Figure 5.1. Process of Concept Derivation

While concept derivation might appear to be a mechanical process, creativity and imagination are required on at least two fronts. First of all, a theorist must select a parent field (F_1) with concepts that bear an analogy to the new field. Seeing an analogous relationship between two fields is not always easy. Frequently, concepts from the natural sciences have been extended into the social and behavioral sciences because they contain rich analogies. For example, concepts such as "system" from biology and "energy" from physics are common in both nursing as well as the social and behavioral sciences. There is no rule, however, about where one may find a rich conceptual perspective for concept derivation. Insight of the theorist is needed.

Second, creativity and imagination are needed in redefining the concepts when they are transposed into a new field. Redefining is more than merely assigning a slightly modified definition to a word. The type of redefinition that occurs in productive concept derivation requires that the concepts be linked to the new field (F_2) by definitions that result in truly innovative and meaningful ways of looking at phenomena in F_2. Perhaps one of the most innovative and meaningful uses of concept derivation results when a new taxonomy or typology of phenomena in F_2 is derived. A new taxonomy or typology provides not only a new vocabulary for classifying phenomena in F_2, but, more important, new ways of looking at F_2. An especially interesting typology in nursing was derived by Roy (Roy & Roberts, 1981, p. 55). Using Helson's concepts of focal, contextual, and residual stimuli from psychophysics, Roy redefined these concepts within nursing to form a typology of factors related to adaptation levels of persons (Roy & Roberts, 1981, pp. 53–55). This derivation process is presented in Figure 5.2.

Concept derivation is not the same as applying a concept in unchanged form to a phenomenon where it has not been previously used. For example, assume that the concept "role change" has not been previously applied to the transition from in-hospital patient to out-patient. Assume further that the concept "role change" may be applied to the transition in patient status without any change in the meaning of the concept of role change. The application of that con-

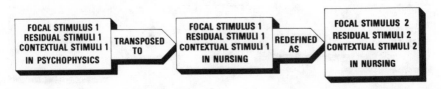

Figure 5.2. Concept Derivation from Helson's to Roy's Concepts

cept to transition in patient status may be scientifically interesting. It is not, however, a true case of concept derivation because role change as a concept was not redefined. Rather role change was simply applied to a new phenomenon to which it already had relevance and meaning. Role change thus was not used as a metaphor or analogy, but rather its meaning was left intact. In true concept derivation more is required than simply applying an existing concept to a phenomenon. The meaning of the concept must be developed and changed to fit a new phenomenon.

PURPOSE AND USES

The purpose of concept derivation is to generate new ways of thinking about and looking at some phenomenon. It provides a new vocabulary for studying an area of interest by relying on an analogous or metaphorical relationship between two phenomena: one defined and known, one undefined and unknown. By relying on a parent field (F_1) for ways of talking about and understanding another (F_2), the concept development process can be accelerated compared to slower methods such as concept synthesis, in which observations and data play a large part in concept development.

Concept derivation is useful in two particular situations: (1) in fields or areas in which no concept development has yet occurred, and (2) in fields in which extant concepts have been available for some time but have contributed little to practical or theoretical growth in the field.

Nurses frequently encounter new situations in which little existing conceptual work has been done; for example, dealing with patients in their ninth decade who have no living relatives except grandchildren and great-grandchildren. Existing concepts about parent–adult child relationships may simply not apply to understanding these skipped-generational family relationships in a highly mobile society. Concept derivation can be useful in constructing new concepts needed to describe the three-generational span of family relationships.

Existing concepts simply may become outmoded, warranting new ways of classifying the phenomena in a field. For example, the traditional concepts that divided areas of nursing practice into medical, surgical, obstetrical, pediatric, and psychiatric nursing are less relevant today than in the past. These divisions are less useful now as more and more is known about how developmental, environmental, and psychological factors interact with the human body to produce disease and health in people. Thus, a new perspective for classifying nursing specialties is needed. Concept derivation can be helpful in constructing a more relevant classification system.

PROCEDURES FOR CONCEPT DERIVATION

There are four basic steps in the concept derivation strategy. While some of these steps in actual practice may occur simultaneously, we present them in logical sequence here to facilitate clarity. Further, users of this strategy may find as they proceed that they need to return to preceding steps to clarify or validate their work at an earlier step. This is especially likely to happen as users move from an orientation phase, that is, getting familiar with their topic of interest, to the intense working phase. We underscore these points so that readers are not misled. While concept derivation is an efficient strategy for concept development, to carry it out adequately is not necessarily a quick, mechanical process.

1. The first step in concept derivation is to become thoroughly familiar with existing literature on one's topic. This involves not only reading that literature but critiquing the level and usefulness of existing concept development found there. If the existing literature on one's topic of interest is lacking in relevant concepts, or if concepts exist but they have ceased to stimulate growth of understanding about the topic, then concept derivation may be suitable as a theory development strategy.
2. Search other fields for new ways of looking at the topic of interest. Read widely in both related and dissimilar fields. Because one cannot know in advance exactly where the most fruitful analogies will be found, it is advisable to begin by casting a broad net at first. From a practical standpoint, it is important not to rush this step, because frequently the analogies surface or become apparent at unexpected times and places. Since this step relies to some extent on creative insight, it can be facilitated by maintaining a relaxed, patient attitude and not trying to force an immediate solution.
3. Select a parent concept or set of concepts from another field to use in the derivation process. The parent-field concepts should offer a new and insightful way of viewing the topic of interest. For example, when one of us was puzzled by some unexpected findings about inconsistencies within mothers, the field of submarine design was a useful analogy for understanding the "compartmentalizing" that seemed at work.
4. Redefine the concept or set of concepts from the parent field in

terms of the topic of interest. In the example mentioned in the step above, the maternal inconsistencies were conceptualized as the "submarine syndrome," which was defined as closing off areas in which a mother was impaired so that these did not incapacitate the other parenting functions, that is, analogous to efforts to prevent sinking the submarine. If a *set* of concepts is being redefined in terms of the topic of interest, these can provide a preliminary taxonomy for describing the basic types that comprise the topic of interest. Once a preliminary set of definitions has been made, check these out with colleagues familiar with the topic of interest. Any constructive criticism received, while momentarily painful, can be very helpful in further refining the initial work. Be sure to give yourself a pat on the back at this point!

The process of concept derivation will be illustrated by presenting an example from the field of human development. The example will trace Sameroff's work on levels of parental thinking about the parent-child relationship (Sameroff, 1980, pp. 348–352).

Sameroff, an expert in child development, began with a working familiarity of literature on human development and family relationships. Sameroff was searching for a new way of understanding parental thought processes that might explain differences in parental childrearing behaviors. He reviewed existing concepts relevant to understanding parental thinking: parental attitudes and expectations and social norms. These concepts in themselves provided only limited ways of understanding parental thinking. In sum, a new perspective was needed. Sameroff was interested in "the level of abstraction utilized by parents to understand development" (p. 349). Citing Piaget, he identified an analogy between cognitive development in children and parental thinking:

> Research on the cognitive development of the child has shown that the infant must go through a number of stages before achieving the logical thought processes that characterize adulthood. Similarly, parents may use different levels in thinking about their relationship with the child (p. 349).

Using Piaget's four stages of cognitive development (sensorimotor, preoperational, concrete operational, and formal operational), Sameroff proposed by analogy four levels of parental thinking. Briefly, at the sensorimotor stage, cognition is tied to actions with learning being rooted in the senses and manipulation. With passage into the next stage, the preoperational, the child uses images and symbols in addition to actions in cognitive processes, but objects are understood in terms of single methods of classification, for example, size. Advancing to the concrete operational stage allows the child to think in terms of logical operations or rules, such as equivalence and serialization, for example, grouping objects in a series by size. In the final stage, formal operations, the child's logical operations are not limited to the real. Rather, hypotheses of abstract possibilities may be proposed and evaluated (Mussen et al., 1980; Biehler, 1971).

Sameroff proposed four analogous levels of parental thinking: symbiotic, categorical, compensatory, and perspectivistic (see Figure 5.3). Parents who respond to the child from the symbiotic level act on a here-and-now basis. Parents do not separate the child's or infant's responses from their own actions. At the categorical level parents see themselves as separate from the child. The child's behavior stems from traits or characteristics of the child, for example, the child is stubborn. Parents who view the child from a compensatory level see the child's behavior as age related, for example, the child is stubborn because he or she is a toddler. At the perspectivistic level, parents see the child's behavior "as stemming from individual experiences in specific environments. If those experiences had been different, the child's characteristics would be different" (Sameroff, 1980, p. 352). Interestingly, Sameroff found that the majority of parents he studied functioned at the categorical level.

In looking back at Sameroff's process, his expertise in the child development field allowed him to complete the first two steps of concept derivation with ease. He knew the literature and was able to critique the utility of existing concepts in the field. This expertise also made readily available to him alternative perspectives needed in deriving concepts about parental thinking levels and also led to selecting Piaget's work as most promising. He then proceeded to flesh out the parental levels of thinking that were analogous to Piaget's stages. In the final step of concept derivation, Sameroff transposed Piaget's concepts and redefined them in ways relevant to parental thinking. He also took the liberty of renaming or creating new labels

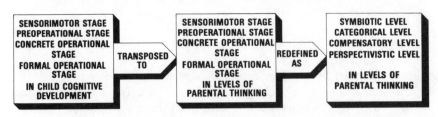

Figure 5.3. Concept Derivation from Piaget's to Sameroff's Concepts

for Piaget's four stages so that the terms in his new framework better fit the parenting phenomenon.

Since the purpose of this book is to describe strategies of theory development rather than those of theory evaluation, we will not judge the scientific merit of Sameroff's work. That may be left to others better qualified. We will point out, however, that Sameroff's use of concept derivation provides a new and interesting framework for practitioners and researchers to consider in studying parent-child relationships.

In applying concept derivation to nursing, several things should be kept in mind. First, since the concerns of nurses overlap with those of other health professions, the first step of concept derivation need not be limited to nursing literature. Medical, educational, developmental, and social work literature, to mention only a few, may be relevant to developing a sense of extant concepts about the topic of interest. Should concepts from these related fields seem adequate, there is no need to proceed any farther. In turn, if an extensive search of literature shows that related fields have not attended to the topic of interest, or if the conceptual work elsewhere seems limited, then concept derivation in nursing may benefit these other fields as well.

Second, as noted earlier, there is no rule about where to look for rich analogies or metaphors for nursing phenomena. The natural sciences (physics, zoology, chemistry) and behavioral sciences as well as applied areas such as law, engineering, and education may be considered. Discussions with nursing colleagues as well as experts in other fields may be useful in identifying potentially useful parent fields from which to derive concepts.

Third, in selecting a promising set of concepts from which to derive concepts for nursing phenomena, theorists should not be impatient. Frequently, assimilation or incubation time is needed to see the fit between two fields of study. This type of insight typically comes in "a flash" that may be preceded by a period of frustrating lack of progress.

Finally, the last step of concept derivation, redefining the concepts in terms of the phenomena in the field of interest, may be laborious. Definitions may need to be redone several times before a final satisfactory outcome is achieved. Setting aside the work for brief periods of time may be helpful in producing the new and creative perspective desired. Critically judging the merits of one's work prematurely may also stifle creativity. The theorist should remain patient but persistent.

ADVANTAGES AND LIMITATIONS

The main advantage of concept derivation as a strategy is that the theorist does not have to begin from scratch. The use of concepts from another field speeds along the creative process. Indeed, Maccia (1963) has suggested that the perspective concept derivation employs may underlie sources of theory development in general.

There are two limitations to concept derivation as a theory-development strategy. First, although the derived concepts may provide useful labels, concepts alone are limited in their scientific usefulness. In themselves, concepts do not provide explanations, predictions, or control of phenomena. Only relational statements and theories have this potential. Development of concepts, however, can be the first stage in development of statements and theories. Concepts may label the dimensions of a phenomenon, but more is needed to achieve the larger goals of science and practice.

Second, although a concept (C_1) from the parent field (F_1) may be very useful in that field, a concept derived from it (C_2) will not automatically be equally useful. Unfortunately, being well born does not guarantee success. Thus, the scientific utility of a derived concept is unknown until it is tested in practice and research. Uncertainty about the scientific usefulness of new ideas is not limited only to concept derivation as a strategy. There is risk endemic in proposing any new idea. Until ideas are tested, their value remains unknown.

UTILIZING THE RESULTS OF CONCEPT DERIVATION

The concepts developed through the derivation strategy may be used in at least two ways in research and theory development: (1) Derived concepts can provide working concepts for use in clinical work such as nursing diagnosis development; and (2) derived concepts can provide preliminary classification schemes of nursing phenomena for use in further research and theory development. In either of these uses it is important to determine if the concepts derived have empirical validity in the new field. To test the validity of derived diagnostic concepts, readers are referred to the methodology literature in the field of nursing diagnosis (e.g., Gordon & Sweeney, 1979). In applying derived concepts to further research and theory development, concepts should be reassessed for their utility in describing phenomena in ways that further the growth of a field of study and in pulling together the findings of relevant research. Where derived concepts delineate new phenomena in need of systematic measurement, they may be used as the base for tool development [see Waltz et al. (1984) on operationalizing nursing concepts].

In education settings concept derivation can be used as an instructional heuristic. Where new concepts that students have no background in are being introduced, analogs can facilitate concept introduction. Such application of concept derivation requires that useful analogs be available and already known to students.

SUMMARY

In this chapter the strategy of concept derivation has been presented. This strategy employs an analogy or metaphor to transpose concepts from one field of study to another. There are no exact rules for selecting a field from which to derive concepts. Concept derivation is suited to topics of interest in which there is no extant concept development or in which existing concepts have become outmoded. The steps in concept derivation include becoming familiar with and critiquing existing literature on a topic, searching other fields for conceptual perspectives, selecting a promising set of concepts from which to derive new concepts, and then generating new concepts by analogy from the parent field.

Concept derivation may speed up the concept development process. The strategy is limited by the level of theory achieved and the uncertainty about the ultimate usefulness of the derived concepts.

PRACTICE EXERCISES

This practice exercise will let you try out the steps of the concept derivation process. Because it is not feasible to do each step completely, we will assume the results of certain steps to facilitate the exercise.

First, let us assume that you are interested in the topic of nurse-patient communication in primary care settings. Let us assume further that after an extensive review of literature on nurse-patient communication you find that the literature lacks concepts particularly relevant to primary care. After searching the behavioral sciences and finding little that seems promising, you happen to talk with a geographer at a social function. He is discussing the concepts that underlie the design and uses of maps. During the course of the conversation, you see a striking analogy between the map concepts and idea of nurse-patient communication in primary care. You see

TABLE 5.1. TWO EXAMPLES OF DERIVED CONCEPTS

Parent Field: Informational Functions of Maps for Travelers	New Field of Interest: Informational Functions of Primary Care Nurses
Example 1. Parent Concepts	*Example 1. Derived Concepts*
1. Direction	1. Orientation
2. Points of interest	2. Facilities available
3. Alternate routes	3. Alternates for diagnosis and treatment
4. Mileage estimates	4. Duration of care
5. Geographic reference points	5. Reference points for progress
6. Destination	6. Goal of care
Example 2. Parent Concepts and Defining Qualities	*Example 2. Derived Concepts and Defining Qualities*
1. Business travel—for a specific purpose	1. Focused care—care of a specific problem
1.1 Efficient travel pace	1.1 Rapid attention to presenting problem
1.2 Direct route on main thoroughfares	1.2 Focus of attention on presenting problem
1.3 Specific information on access points on route	1.3 Specific information about time and place of treatments
1.4 Reliable accommodations	1.4 Reliable personnel and facilities
1.5 Time frame limited to specific business objective	1.5 Time frame for care determined by presenting problem
2. Pleasure travel—travel for recreation and growth	2. Revitalization care—care for health promotion
2.1 Leisurely pace of travel	2.1 Careful consideration to patient concerns and questions
2.2 Scenic routes	2.2 Attention to overall health status
2.3 Alternate access points for possible side trips	2.3 Information about health promotion alternatives
2.4 Pleasurable accommodations	2.4 Competent and humanistic care
2.5 Time frame negotiable based on wishes	2.5 Time frame negotiated based on health promotion needs and wants

the patient as a "traveler" and the nurse as a source of "travel information" in getting to a "destination."

To do this exercise, take out a map of your state. List the kinds of information the map provides a traveler. List how you use a map as you travel between two cities in your state. List the different reasons you might be traveling and how this might affect what you refer to on the map. Review these lists thoroughly. Now select the key ideas from these lists that seem to you to describe the ways a traveler uses a map to get to a destination. Now think of the patient and nurse in a primary care setting. Transfer your key ideas (i.e., concepts) about the ways a traveler uses a map to the primary care setting. Use these key ideas to think about nurse-patient communication. When you get a "feel" for these key ideas in the primary care setting, jot down short definitions that describe the concepts in terms of nurse-patient communication. Do not worry yet about whether your definitions and concepts make sense. Set your work aside for a while. Look at your key concepts and definitions again. Clarify any fuzzy wording or ideas. Now try out your ideas on some colleagues who will give constructive criticism. From their reactions, further refine your concepts and definitions.

There is no one "right" set of concepts or definitions that you should have derived. If you had had a colleague simultaneously do this same exercise, that person's concepts and definitions would probably be somewhat different from yours. For comparison purposes, two examples of concepts that we derived by this exercise are presented in Table 5.1. In example 2, the defining characteristics of the derived concepts are also provided. You may find that the concepts and definitions that you derived are more interesting than the ones we present!

REFERENCES

Biehler RF: Psychology Applied to Teaching. Boston: Houghton Mifflin, 1971.

Gordon M, Sweeney MA: Methodological problems and issues in identifying and standardizing nursing diagnoses. Adv Nurs Sci 2(1): 1–15, 1979.

Maccia ES: Ways of inquiring. In (ES Maccia, GS Maccia, & RE Jewett, eds.), Construction of Educational Theory Models. Washington, D.C.: Office of Education, U.S. Dept. of Health, Education, and Welfare, Cooperative Research Project No. 1632, 1963, 1–13.

Mussen PH, Conger JJ, Kagan J: Essentials of Child Development and Personality. Philadelphia: Harper & Row, 1980.

Roy C, Roberts SL: Theory Construction in Nursing: An Adaptation Model. Englewood Cliffs, N.J.: Prentice-Hall, 1981.

Sameroff AJ: Issues in early reproductive and caretaking risk: Review and current status. In (DB Sawin, RC Hawkins, LO Walker, JH Penticuff, eds.), Exceptional Infant. Vol. 4. Psychosocial Risks in Infant-Environment Transactions. New York: Brunner/Mazel, 1980, 343–359.

Waltz CF, Strickland OL, Lenz ER: Measurement in Nursing Research. Philadelphia: Davis, 1984, 19–41.

PART III
Statement Development

When is development of statements an important goal of theory development? Actually, much of the working backbone of a science resides in its laws and empirical generalizations, both being forms of scientific statements. In a practice discipline, indeed many of the interventions of practice may be based on relational statements. For example, Barnard (1982) proposed the following statement: "In the presence of internal system instability the environment can provide regulators which assist the human system in reintegrating body processes" (p. 7). Although very abstractly stated, this statement (which Barnard calls a theory) leads to nursing interventions that impose external environmental structuring in order to aid a person in establishing his or her own endogenous structuring where none or only a weak one previously existed. Thus, statement development can be a very important and useful level of theory development for practice. It is especially relevant when a theorist wishes to go beyond the concept (labeling) phase but does not need the comprehensive perspectives offered by a theory.

To determine which statement-development strategy is most suitable to a theorist's purposes, it is essential to assess the "state of the art" of existing knowledge about one's topic of interest. To make this determination, first clearly identify what the topic of interest is. Then read key articles or references that are up to date and capture the main ideas about the topic of interest. If a topic is new, it is likely that available resources will not be very comprehensive. After reading materials carefully, form your judgment about the "state of the art." If the literature is well developed but not research-based, statement analysis

(Chapter 6) may be a useful starting strategy. If the literature primarily contains research findings that need to be integrated, then literary methods of statement synthesis (Chapter 7) may be suitable. Finally, if the existing literature shows the topic of interest to be undeveloped, or if existing literature is simply outmoded and in need of a fresh start, statement synthesis (Chapter 7) or statement derivation (Chapter 8) may be appropriate. In the latter situation, statement synthesis can be undertaken if the theorist has the resources and inclination for collecting and analyzing observations, either qualitatively or quantitatively; if this is not so, statement derivation can be undertaken. While more than one strategy may be fitted to the state of a topical area, it is advisable to select one and use it until it ceases to be useful rather than trying to use two or three strategies simultaneously.

REFERENCES

Barnard KE: The research cycle: Nursing, the profession, the discipline. Proceedings of the 1982 Conference of the Western Society for Research in Nursing. Western Journal of Nursing Research 4(3) 1–12, 1982.

6
Statement
Analysis

DEFINITION AND DESCRIPTION

Statement analysis is a process of examining relational statements to determine in what form they are presented and what relationship the concepts within those statements have to one another. As in all analyses, statement analysis includes the examination of each part and its relationship to each other part and to the whole. Statement analysis focuses on each concept within a statement, the relationship of each concept with each other concept, and the role the statement plays as a whole.

As we have said, there are two types of nonrelational statements used in theory (see Chapter 2). One is what Reynolds (1971) has called an *existence* statement. This type of statement simply identifies a concept or an object and claims its existence. For example, we might say "the phenomenon of a person's subjective feelings is termed the affect." The label "affect" is claimed to exist and is identified by a brief summary statement. Existence statements occur in theories to provide background and explanation prior to positing relationships.

The second type of nonrelational statement in theory is called a *definition*. A definition describes the characteristics of a concept. It may be a theoretical definition—one that is abstract and useful to the theory but with no empirical referents named—or it may be an operational definition, in which the method of measurement is clearly spelled out. Leaving rods and cones out of it for now, let us assume that the concept of "colorblindness" has a theoretical definition that implies visual inability to distinguish accurately between colors. The operational definition of colorblindness, then, might include criteria such as which colors would be included in testing, how many times the test must be run, and how many "wrong" answers constitute failure before "colorblindness" can be said to be present. Definitions are useful in theory because they provide the basis for clear communication between the theorist and the reader/user.

In theory building, statements are usually thought of as relational statements. Each statement describes some type of relationship among the concepts within it. Relational statements are a bit more complex than either existence statements or definitions. Basically they come in several forms that will be discussed individually in the analysis section. Suffice it to say at this point that relational statements may be associational, causal, deterministic, probabilistic, or theoretical (Reynolds, 1971). Relational statements are the skeleton of theory. They are the means by which everything appears to hang together. When they occur singly, they form the basis for research or at least further reflection on the phenomenon in question. When they occur in groups and are not interrelated, they are the stimulus for thinking and exploration to find their linkages. If they occur in groups and are interrelated, they are called "theory."

PURPOSES AND USES

Statement analysis is a way of examining statements in an orderly way in an effort to determine if the statements are useful, informative, and logically correct. It is a rigorous process.

The purposes of statement analysis are (1) to classify statements as to form and (2) to examine the relationship between the concepts. Statement analysis is suited to situations in which one or more statements about a phenomenon exist but have not yet been organized into a theoretical system. The strategy is useful in that it provides the theorist with information about the structure and function of the statements being considered. In addition it is particularly useful because once the statement has been analyzed, any deficiencies in it are obvious and may be corrected or modified.

Statement analysis provides a way of looking at and formalizing theoretical constructions that are already available in the literature or through research. It is also useful when a theorist is building a "new" theory, to carefully analyze the proposed relational statements before subjecting them to the criticism and scrutiny that such a "new" theory invariably generates from the scholarly community.

STEPS IN STATEMENT ANALYSIS

There are seven steps in statement analysis: (1) select the statement(s) to be analyzed; (2) simplify the statement; (3) classify the statement; (4) examine concepts within the statement for definition and validity; (5) specify relationships between concepts by type, sign, and symmetry; (6) examine the logic; and (7) determine testability.

Selecting the Statement

Although the first step appears to be the easiest, it may, in fact, prove very difficult. Selecting a statement to be analyzed involves some commitment to the idea behind the statement. One does not usually choose to do statement analysis without some underlying purpose. Anyone attempting statement analysis should have clearly in mind what reason he or she has for doing so. Perhaps you have some doubt about the statement, or perhaps the idea excites you and you wish to examine the structure for soundness before you refute it or act upon it in some way. In any case, the theorist should have the rationale for analysis clearly in mind before beginning.

The second reason for the difficulty in selecting a statement is the problem that arises in some verbal or written theories: a lack of specificity of relational statements. Theories, especially in the social and behavioral sciences, may be elaborately verbal (Blalock, 1969). On close inspection, however, one may find it very difficult to isolate one single relational statement. It then becomes the task of the analyst to extract or construct simple relational statements from all the verbiage. This exercise requires a great deal of careful reading to be sure one has actually reflected the meaning in the way the original theorist intended. Crosschecking with colleagues or even the original theorist is often a big help when you are confronted by such a problem.

The third consideration in selecting a statement for analysis is that it be relevant. That is, it is far better to select a prominent or major statement in a theory than to select an insignificant one. To tell the difference in major and minor statements, examine the statement's breadth. A major statement will yield more information to the analyst than a minor one will. In addition, if the major statement has validity, the likelihood increases that the minor one does too.

Simplify the Statement If Necessary

This step is only necessary if one of two things occurs. The first is the problem of the elaborate verbal model that must be reduced to manageable statements. The second problem is complexity, which may occur in theories in which one concept may be linked to several others at the same time. When this happens, it simplifies analysis to break the concept linkages into several shorter, more manageable statements. Assume a statement could be diagrammed as the one in Figure 6.1. It is clear that the analyst might find his or her job much easier to handle if the formulation looked more like the one in Figure 6.2. The analyst now has four simple discreet relationships to examine instead of one set of complex relationships. It is also clear, however, that great care must be exercised when doing this or relationships may be overlooked or misconstrued.

Classify the Statement

When we speak of the classification of a statement we are examining the use of the statement within the theory. There are three basic classifications of statements: (1) existence statements, (2) definitions, and (3) relational statements.

Existence statements claim existence for concepts (Reynolds, 1971). The statement "That object is called a refrigerator" is an existence statement. Existence statements are not definitions and thus do not describe characteristics of the concept. They simply assert that something is so. Existence statements can be accurate or inaccurate. If the object in our example is really a dishwasher then the statement is inaccurate. If the object in the statement corresponds to reality (it *is* a refrigerator) then the statement is accurate.

Definitions have three subforms—descriptive, stipulative, and operational (Hempel, 1966). A descriptive definition describes the accepted meaning for a term already in use. It describes the term in other terms that are already understood by the reader. It generally can be considered accurate.

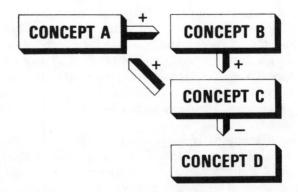

Figure 6.1. A Complicated Statement. See Figure 6.2 for Simplification.

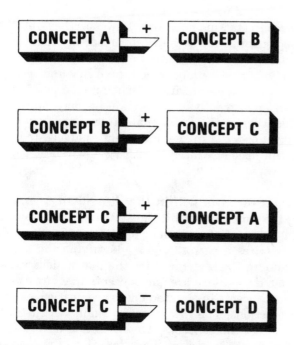

Figure 6.2. The Statement in Figure 6.1 Broken Down into Several Shorter More Manageable Statements

A stipulative definition, on the other hand, describes the term in such a way that it has a very specific use within the theory; a use that is not always the same as the general meaning of the term. These definitions cannot be considered either accurate or inaccurate because they are specifically formulated *only* for use in the way the author of the theory has decreed.

For example, a descriptive definition of "kitten" might read "A kitten is the biological offspring of an adult female cat." A stipulative definition of "kitten," however, might read "For the purpose of this study, a kitten shall be defined as any healthy female offspring of a healthy female cat that is less than eight weeks old."

A stipulative definition is not the same as an operational definition. An operational definition includes the specific means for measuring or testing each scientific term within it. An operational definition must be so precise that it can be used repetitively by different scientists and still obtain objective results. In our definition of "kitten," for instance, the operational definition might be "For the purposes of this study, a kitten shall be any healthy offspring of a healthy female cat weighing between 4 and 12 ounces and no less than 3 days or more than 12 days old."

A *relational* statement is one that specifies relationships between concepts. It may be so well supported empirically and logically
that it functions as a law or an axiom within the theory. It may be
less well supported by data or logic than a law and serve as a proposition or empirical generalization. Or it may be any hypothesis that
is as yet unsupported by data even if it may appear reasonable
logically. Identifying the relational statements is very important
when you get to Step 5 in the statement analysis. It is that step in
which you will specify exactly which *type* of relationship the statement exemplifies.

Examine the Concepts within the Statement

Identifying the concepts within the statement to be analyzed is perhaps the easiest part of statement analysis. It is the examination of
them that requires a certain rigor. Identifying the concepts simply
involves scanning the statement for the major ideas expressed in it.
The labels for these ideas are the concepts that must be examined.

After the concepts in a statement are identified, examining them
involves two actions. The first is to determine the definitions of the
terms that reflect the concepts. The definition should reflect all the
critical defining attributes or characteristics of the concept so that
everyone who reads the theory will know precisely how the theorist
intends the term to be used. (For a discussion of determining defining attributes for a concept, see Chapter 3.) If the concept is not
adequately defined, can its meaning be determined from the context
of the theoretical formulation? If so, the analyst should use this
material to help formulate additions to the definition that will aid
the analysis and even perhaps help refine the theory. If not, then the
analyst must simply state that the concepts are inadequately defined
for the purpose of analysis.

The second step in the examination of concepts in a statement is
to determine if the concepts *as they are defined* are theoretically
valid. This process is a bit like determining construct validity in
research. That is, the analyst attempts to determine whether the
concepts as they are defined accurately reflect the general semantic
usage for that concept. This process involves a brief overview of the
relevant literature that concerns the concept being considered. If the
concept is being used in the same ways as it has previously been used
in the literature and the definition reflects it, the concept may be
considered valid. In addition, if the theorist has conducted a careful
concept analysis, the concept is considered valid even if it does not
reflect the relevant literature but goes beyond traditional usage. The
concept may be more valid, in fact, than a concept defined by tradition alone.

Specify Relationships by Type, Sign, and Symmetry

Type. The assessment of a relational statement for type, sign, and symmetry is for the purpose of determining its function. Several types of relational statements may occur. These are causal, probabilistic, concurrent, conditional, time-order, necessary, and sufficient types of statements (Hardy, 1974). We shall consider each type briefly and give an example of each. For the purposes of clarity and simplicity, we are assuming that all relational statements are linear until proven otherwise. (Statement analysis can often provide the clue to curvilinear relationships. If you can't classify a statement or determine its sign, it may express a nonlinear relationship.)

The causal statement is one in which the first concept is said to be the "cause" of the other. Causal statements are generally deduced from laws. There are few causal statements in the social and behavioral sciences primarily because there are so many intervening variables that influence causation. There are more in the physical sciences. For example, the statement "Raising the temperature of a gas held under constant pressure will increase its volume" is a causal statement. It asserts that some event (raising the temperature of a gas under pressure) causes another event (increased gas volume). This is the simplest form of causal statement although there are more complex ones involving several causal events for one phenomenon. Causal statements are difficult to find, especially in beginning attempts at theory construction, because the caused event must *always* happen if the causal event or events occur.

It is often helpful to use symbols for the concepts in statements so that you don't become confused by the content of the concepts during analysis. Using the symbols G_p for gas under pressure, T for temperature, and GV for gas volume, you can diagram the statement thus:

$$\text{If } \uparrow T \rightarrow G_p \text{ then always } \uparrow GV.$$

If the event (GV) always occurs, it can be labeled a causal statement.

If the event only occurs some of the time or even most of the time, but not *all* of the time, the statement is called probabilistic. Probabilistic statements are usually derived from statistical data. They assert that if one event occurs, the second event probably will also. An excellent example of a probabilistic statement is that cigarette smoking (CS) is highly likely to lead to lung cancer (LC). There is no direct causality in this statement since everyone who smokes does not acquire lung cancer. But the *probability* of acquiring lung cancer is increased significantly in the presence of cigarette smoking. Probabilistic relationships, if diagrammed, might look like this:

If $CS \rightarrow$ then probably LC.

Concurrent relationships demonstrate that if event A occurs, event B also occurs. There may or may not be any correlation or causation between the two events—they simply exist together. An example of this kind of statement might be "A low level of educational preparation and a low income often occur together." The statement does not infer that little education *causes* poverty or even that the two are correlated. Another example can be found in Muhlenkamp and Parsons' study of nurses (1972) and is confirmed in Kaiser and Bickle's study (1980). These authors found that nurses have personality characteristics that are highly feminine rather than masculine. This is a good example of a concurrent statement. It simply asserts that nurses (N) and feminine personality (FP) characteristics occur together. It makes no other claim. A diagram of this statement would be:

If N, also FP.

A conditional statement is one that demonstrates a relationship between two concepts or events but that requires the presence of a third concept or event before the relationship can come about. A good example of a conditional statement is one found in a study by Reichert and Fuller on the effects of sodium bicarbonate on intraventricular hemorrhage in premature infants (1980). Their statement indicates that sodium bicarbonate ($NaHCO_3$) can be given to correct acidosis in premature infants with respiratory distress without the occurrence of intraventricular hemorrhage (IVH) but only if given in conservative doses (CD) and over a 15- to 30-minute time period (TTP). This can be simplistically diagrammed as:

If $NaHCO_3$, then no IVH, but only if CD and TTP.

Time-ordered statements are those that indicate that some amount of time intervenes between the first concept or event and the second. An example of a time-ordered statement might be one that indicates that if a person experiences numerous stressful life events (SLE) within a year the likelihood of that person becoming ill (I) is quite high (Holmes & Rahe, 1968; Rahe, 1972). This relationship is time-ordered because time passes between the first episodes of stress and the resultant illness. This statement can be diagrammed like this:

If *SLE*, then later *I*.

A necessary relationship is shown by a statement that indicates that one and only one concept or event can lead to the second concept or event. These necessary relationships function very much as differential diagnoses do in medicine. That is, a patient can be positively said to have cancer, for instance, if and only if there is a pathologist's report of malignant cells on biopsy. In the same way, relationships among concepts may only occur under certain conditions. An example from nursing might be a statement relating to stress and adaptation. Both Roy's (1976) and Neuman's (1980) models of nursing have stated that adaptation (*A*) occurs as a response to stressors (*S*). Stressors then become *necessary* before adaptation can occur. The diagram would look like this:

If and only if *S*, then *A*.

Sufficient relationships are reflected in statements in which the first concept or event and the second concept or event are related regardless of anything else. Using the stressor/adaptation idea above, we can see that if stressors occur then adaptation will begin in the person whether or not she or he wills it and whether or not someone intervenes to help. In other words, the presence of the first concept guarantees the presence of the second concept. A sufficient relationship could be diagrammed like this:

If *S*, then *A* regardless of anything else.

Sign. Determining the sign of relationships is reasonably easy. Signs generally fall into one of three categories: positive, negative, or unknown (Mullins, 1971; Reynolds, 1971). The rule of thumb is that if the concepts vary in the same direction, that is, as one increases or decreases so does the other, then the relationship is positive. If one concept increases while the other decreases, the relationship is said to be negative. If you have no information about the way the concepts vary, the relationship is unknown. Below are three probabilistic statements and one inferred statement from the first three with their relationships drawn to help you see how this is done.

When members of a group become anxious (*A*), hostility (*H*) increases.

$$A \overset{+}{\rightarrow} H$$

Hostility is related to a decrease in group cohesiveness (*GC*).

$$H \rightleftharpoons GC$$

Creativity (C) decreases as anxiety increases in groups.

$$A \rightleftharpoons C$$

Inferred: Anxiety has a negative impact on group cohesiveness.

$$A \rightleftharpoons GC$$

This inferred statement was derived logically from the first two statements. Since both A and GC are related to H, they are therefore related to each other.

What we cannot tell from these four statements is what effect creativity and group cohesiveness have on each other. So that might look like this:

$$C \_ \underline{?} \_ GC$$

Symmetry. Relationships can be symmetrical or asymmetrical (Blalock, 1969). So far, all our examples have been asymmetrical, that is, one-direction relationships. In asymmetrical statements, the relationship only goes from one concept to the next but is never reciprocated. There are many examples of asymmetrical relationships in our discussions. One example is the statement above that anxiety is negatively related to group cohesiveness. If the relationship is a two-way relationship in which each concept affects the other, it is considered symmetrical. An example of a symmetrical statement might be one from research done by one of us on maternal attachment behaviors (Avant, 1981). High attachment scores (At) were associated with low anxiety (Ax) scores and high anxiety scores were associated with low attachment scores in primiparous women. This relationship can be diagrammed like this:

$$At \rightleftharpoons Ax$$

Examine the Logic
The logic of a single statement can be examined for origin, reasonableness, and adequacy. When examining the origin of a statement, ask yourself whether the statement is constructed deductively, that is, from a more general law, or inductively, from observation or available data. If the statement is deductive in origin, its logic should be adequate since a conclusion in a deductive argument cannot be false if the premises are true. If the statement is inductive, its logic cannot

be judged except by the amount of empirical support it has and by comparison to existing knowledge (Hempel, 1966). If it has strong support in both empirical testing and in agreement with existing literature, its logic is probably adequate. The logic can also be determined by examining the relationships of the concepts to each other. If the relationship cannot be classified by type, sign, or symmetry, there may be a logical flaw.

Comparison to existing knowledge is also used in determining the reasonableness of a statement. One simply asks if this statement seems reasonable given what we already know on the subject. If it makes sense in the light of existing knowledge, it is reasonable.

Determining adequacy of a single statement is more difficult than determining adequacy of a theory since we cannot construct matrices or models to demonstrate where logical gaps may occur. It is possible, however, to draw a simple diagram as we have done in the previous section labeling the concepts by letters or numbers and determining types and signs that are relevant. If you are unable to do any one of the three, there is some fault in the statement.

Determine Testability
The final step in a statement analysis is to determine if the statement is empirically testable. In this step of the analysis you must determine whether or not there are operational measures that can be used in the "real world" to obtain data that will support or refute the statement. It is at this point that the analyst will run up against the situation Hempel calls "testability-in-principle." Basically, this is a statement that *could* be tested empirically if the tools were available to measure the concepts; but they are not available (Hempel, 1966). He considers these statements equally useful in theory construction as the actually empirically testable statements. Since so many of our concepts in nursing may lack the instruments to measure them, we feel that the criterion of testability can be met if a statement is either testable-in-principle or actually testable.

This is not to imply, however, that all statements are therefore testable. In order for a statement to meet the criterion of testability it must render some test implications. That is, one should be able to say "If I tested this under the specified conditions, then the outcome hypothesized should actually happen." A relatively "new" statement might render fewer testable ideas than one that has more age and support, but if it is testable at all, it meets the criterion. Any statement that cannot produce one testable idea or that is constructed in such a way that the concepts have vague meanings cannot meet the criterion of testability until modified.

ADVANTAGES AND LIMITATIONS

Statement analysis has several advantages. The primary advantage is that it provides a systematic way of examining the relationships between concepts. In addition, it assists the theorist in examining the structure and function of statements. But perhaps the most important function of statement analysis is that when you are thinking carefully and systematically about the linkages between concepts, you may discover other linkages or relationships that are important to the final theoretical formulations. In just such analysis situations have many scientists "happened on to" important theoretical ideas as if by accident.

The limitations of statement analysis are that it is often difficult to analyze just one statement if it is part of a theoretical whole. Removing the statement from its context can often result in loss of valuable information, and the analysis is hindered. In addition, determining the logic of a statement is often more difficult when it is removed from the theory. The final limitation of the statement analysis process is that it does take a little time and it is rigorous. This is only a limitation as it applies to the theorist, however, since it is this very rigorousness and time taking that are ultimately so valuable in assessing statements.

UTILIZING THE RESULTS OF STATEMENT ANALYSIS

Statement analysis formalizes statements so that their underlying structures and functions are made explicit. But what does one do with the resulting information? It can be used in a variety of different ways in education, practice, research, and theory development.

In education, analyzed statements can be used as springboards for discussion. Discussions can include ideas about which concepts were clear, which ones were related to each other, and how, or what, inconsistencies were discovered. The amount of empirical evidence for or against the statement can be examined and used as the basis for designing classroom activities such as proposing research studies that would produce either more evidence for the statement or more evidence against the statement. The amount of empirical evidence could also be used to launch a discussion about the efficacy of the statement to guide clinical practice. Another use for statement analysis in education might be to have a faculty interest group discuss the issues raised from analyzing several similar statements or several statements about the same topic of interest. This discussion could lead to curriculum changes or to faculty research projects.

In practice, statement analysis can guide clinicians in the judicious use of research findings. Knowing whether or not a statement is associational, causal, or time ordered can help in decisions about when to use the statement and under what conditions. Certain nursing diagnoses may be considered or certain nursing interventions chosen as a result of the statement analysis that might not have been considered previously by the nurse. In addition, faced with the choice of two potential interventions, statement analysis would provide the nurse with knowledge of which has the most empirical support, thus leading to a more educated decision on her part.

In research, statement analysis provides fruitful information about what the next steps in a research program are. Inconsistencies, unclear definitions, and gaps in knowledge become apparent. These provide direction for planning concept analyses, reformulating ideas, or proposing new hypotheses to test.

In theory development, statement analysis allows the theorist to see where the problems in a statement are and to take the appropriate next step. Do concepts need clarifying? Are there inconsistencies? If so, the theorist can plan strategies for dealing with these issues. If the analysis has demonstrated that the statement is sound, the theorist can begin to look for additional concepts and linkages to add to what is already known. This is how theories are built—one step at a time.

SUMMARY

We have said that statement analysis is a process of systematically examining the relationships between concepts. There are seven steps involved: selecting the statement; simplifying it if necessary; classifying it; examining the concepts for definition and validity; specifying relationships by type, sign, and symmetry; examining the logic; and determining the testability.

The process of statement analysis provides useful information for the theorist in that once the statement has been analyzed, any deficiencies in the statement are clear and may be corrected. In addition, the process of thinking aloud (or in writing) about two or more concepts often generates additional statements either by deduction or by serendipity that are valuable additions to future theoretical formulations. We shall see how this is often done in the next two chapters on statement synthesis and statement derivation.

PRACTICE EXERCISES

Below are several statements from a study of faculty attitudes (Ruiz, 1981).

A. Classify each statement as either
   a. Relational statement
   b. Descriptive definition
   c. Stipulative definition
   d. Operational definition
   1. Ethnocentrism means ethnic narrow-mindedness.
   2. Dogmatism shall be defined as close-mindedness.
   3. Intolerance of ambiguity and dogmatism are the two factors underlying ethnocentrism for this study.
   4. Faculty who are highly dogmatic view patients with different ethnocultural backgrounds as annoying and superstitious.
   5. Faculty who have high ethnocentrism scores have negative attitudes toward culturally different patients.
B. Using statement 4, simplify it into two statements and diagram them.
C. Using statements 4 and 5, examine the concepts and specify the relationships by type, sign, and symmetry. Determine the logic and testability of each.

Answers:

A. 1. b, 2. c, 3. d, 4. a, 5. a
B. **1.** Dogmatic faculty (*DF*) view patients with differing ethnocultural (*DEB*) backgrounds as annoying (*A*):

   If *DF*, then *A*, but only if *DEB*.

   2. Dogmatic faculty (*DF*) view patients with differing ethnocultural backgrounds (*DEB*) as superstitious (*S*):

   If *DF*, then *S*, but only if *DEB*.

C. Statement 4 can be diagrammed as $DF \rightleftharpoons DEB$
   Statement 5 as ethnocentric faculty (*EF*) $\rightleftharpoons$ attitudes toward culturally different patients (*ACDB*) or $EF \rightleftharpoons ACDB$.

   Both statements are probabilistic since they are drawn from statistical data and statement 4 as it is diagrammed in Practice Exercise B is conditional. Both statements are asymmetrical. The signs are negative since less dogmatic faculty had higher views of ethnocentric patients.

Some of the concepts from statements 4 and 5, such as "patient," "faculty," "ethnocultural background," "annoying," and "superstitious," are undefined. If these concepts were intended to be used in their common language meanings, the author should state that clearly. Otherwise each should be defined. The two concepts that were defined, "ethnocentrism" and "dogmatism," are given only in vague, equally undefined terms in this exercise. (They were operationally defined in the actual study.) The concept of "intolerance of ambiguity" is not defined but is used as part of an operational definition. This is clearly to be avoided. None of the concept definitions are unambiguous.

The statements are logical. They are testable only if better concept definitions are constructed so that operational measures can be found for them. Only when there are careful operational definitions that reflect the theoretical definitions can it be said that the concepts are measurable or the statement testable.

REFERENCES

Avant K: Anxiety as a potential factor affecting maternal attachment. JOGN 10(6): 416–420, 1981.

Blalock H, Jr: Theory Construction: From Verbal to Mathematical Formulations. Englewood Cliffs, N.J.: Prentice-Hall, 1969.

Hardy M: Theories: Components, development, and evaluation. Nurs Res 23: 100–126, 1974.

Hardy M (ed.): Theoretical Foundations for Nursing. New York: MSS Information Corporation, 1973.

Hempel C: Philosophy of Science. Englewood Cliffs, N.J.: Prentice-Hall, 1966.

Holmes R, Rahe R: The social readjustment rating scale. J Psychosom Res 11: 213, 1968.

Kaiser J, Bickle I: Attitude change as a motivational factor in producing behavior change related to implementing primary nursing. Nurs Res 19(5): 290–300, 1980.

Muhlenkamp A, Parsons J: Characteristics of nurses: An overview of recent research published in a nursing research periodical. J Vocational Behav 2: 261–273, 1972.

Mullins N: The Art of Theory: Construction and Use. New York: Harper & Row, 1971.

Neuman B: The Betty Neuman health-care systems model. In (JP Riehl & C Roy, eds.), Conceptual Models for Nursing Practice. 2d ed. New York: Appleton-Century-Crofts, 1980.

Rahe R: Subject's recent life changes and their near future illness susceptibility. Adv Psychosom Med 8: 2–19, 1972.

Reichert E, Fuller P: Relationship of sodium bicarbonate to intraventricular hemorrhage in premature infants with respiratory distress syndrome. Nurs Res 29(6): 357–361, 1980.

Reynolds P: A Primer in Theory Construction. Indianapolis: Bobbs-Merrill, 1971.

Roy C: Introduction to Nursing: An Adaptation Model. Englewood Cliffs, N.J.: Prentice-Hall, 1976.

Ruiz M: Open-closed mindedness, intolerance of ambiguity and nursing faculty attitudes toward culturally different patients. Nurs Res 30(3): 177–181, 1981.

ADDITIONAL READINGS

Greenwood D: The Nature of Science and Other Essays. New York: Philosophical Library, 1959.

Hage J: Techniques and Problems of Theory Construction in Sociology. New York: John Wiley & Sons, 1972.

Lerner D (ed.): Parts and Wholes. New York: Free Press of Glencoe, 1963.

Pasch A: Experience and the Analytic: A Reconsideration of Empiricism. Chicago: Univ. of Chicago Press, 1958.

Zetterberg HL: On Theory and Verification in Sociology. 3rd ed. New York: Bedminster Press, 1965.

7
Statement Synthesis

DEFINITION AND DESCRIPTION

Statement synthesis is a strategy that is aimed at specifying relationships between two or more concepts based on evidence. The evidence may come from various sources: (1) direct clinical observations of individuals, (2) statistical information collected from large numbers of people, or (3) library materials reporting completed research. Logically, statement synthesis involves two operations: (1) moving from observations to inferences and then (2) generalizing from specific inferences to more abstract ones.

In the first source of evidence, a thoughtful series of observations may be the basis of interrelating concepts. For example, suppose a nurse-clinician noticed that elderly patients were more cooperative when certain types of interview approaches were used with them. The nurse might state the relationship noted as follows: Elderly patients' cooperativeness is increased if they are encouraged to talk about their life events. In stating this relationship based on her or his own clinical observations, the nurse has taken an important step in statement construction. While an observation based on a very small number of patients is only suggestive that the relationship may also be found among other groups of elderly patients, the observation nonetheless may be useful in directing further theory building.

The second source of evidence, by contrast, uses machine or computer technology to compress many individual observations or measurements of patients into one or more quantitative indices, such as correlation coefficients, before statement synthesis can be done. In this situation, statement synthesis permits relationships expressed in numerical form to be translated into verbal or linguistic form. For example, suppose a correlation of 0.50 was found to exist between cigarette smoking and occurrence of a certain type of cancer, W, in humans. Other things being equal, one way this statistical information could be interpreted is, cigarette smoking is related to form W of cancer in humans. Statistically based statement synthesis such as this can be applied to both descriptive research and experimental research studies.

Finally, if a theorist is interested in constructing statements about a topic on which much research has already been done, still another source of evidence is available, published documents. For example, one might do a library search of research literature to locate factors that affect the success of patient education programs and the benefits that result from patient education. A search of literature might begin by cataloging relationships between variables. Relationships would then be further organized and combined to obtain clear and general statements of relationships between concepts. Because some relationships will be found repeatedly in studies, while others will be found on only one or two occasions, statements may be grouped according to how much support or evidence is available for each statement.

From these introductory descriptions of various forms of statement synthesis, one can see that this strategy consists of multiple and varied methods. The desired outcome of these diverse methods, however, is the same: the clear statement of relationships between two or more concepts. Further, the theorist using statement synthesis pulls together, organizes, or extracts patterns of relationship from information gathered in reality—the outside world. Thus, observations and other methods of scientific measurement, for example, interviews and machine readings, are essential to the process of statement synthesis. Unlike other statement-development strategies, statement synthesis requires empirical evidence in some form.

Knowledge of statistics is not essential for each method of statement synthesis. Familiarity with statistical methods is an indispensable tool, however, where large amounts of quantifiable information are collected. Statistical methods may be useful in collapsing large amounts of gathered information into more interpretable form. Readers should not confuse statistics with statement synthesis. Statistical methods are only adjuncts to the process of specifying relationships between concepts in the field of interest. Information about reality is condensed by statistical procedures.

Because obtaining maximum benefit from this chapter requires knowledge of introductory statistics, readers may wish to assess their readiness for the statistical material included here by completing the pretest located at the end of this chapter. For interested readers, several introductory statistical texts are listed at the end of this chapter.

PURPOSE AND USES

The purpose of statement synthesis is to develop from observation of phenomena one or more statements about relationships that exist between those phenomena. As indicated earlier, the observations may be made directly by the theorist or may be drawn from the literature. Further, where large numbers of observations or measurements are made, these may be treated statistically to compress the information contained in the large data set and put them in a more interpretable form.

Data or observations may be used to develop as well as to test hypotheses. These two uses, while quite distinct, often employ similar techniques particularly in statistically based statement synthesis. This similarity leads to several difficulties. Theorists may needlessly apply rules for justification to a discovery context (see Chapter 1). For example, statistical results with a probability level slightly greater than .05 may be disregarded even though the finding makes sense conceptually.

In turn, theorists may discover certain relationships among phenomena using a loose pragmatic research design and then treat the "discovery" as if it were a well-proven fact. As noted in Chapter 1, it is preferable, as a general rule, to keep the contexts of justification and discovery as distinct as possible. Where data are used to extract relational statements (context of discovery), these same data should not be used again to claim the statements have been "tested" (context of justification). Another independent data set should be used in an attempt to confirm or cross-validate the original findings. Similarly, rigorous testing of hypotheses (context of justification) may be followed by further atheoretical analyses or "massaging" of the data (context of discovery). The latter, while important, does not carry the same evidential status as the former types of analysis.

Where evidence is used for statement synthesis (context of discovery), it should be analyzed in ways that facilitate discovery. This may necessitate altering canons or conventions such as traditional probability levels in order to construct statements that meaningfully reflect relationships inherent in data or observations. Such flexibility may be wise and appropriate in order to maximally exploit information collected about a phenomenon in a discovery context. These same liberties exercised in a justificatory context would probably be seriously frowned upon by responsible scientists. In the interim between discovery and testing operations, many refinements in measurement and conceptualization occur that permit crude "discovery" observations to be more suitably and rigorously tested.

In choosing statement synthesis as a strategy for theory construction, theorists should consider that it is especially suited to situations in which one of the following is true: (1) There is no conceptual or empirical work done to describe a topic of interest, but a series of observations can be made readily to establish some of the parameters (empirical qualities) of the phenomenon; (2) there are several concepts in use in an ، rea of interest, but evidence is needed to clarify how the concepts may be interrelated; (3) there are several published research studies on a phenomenon of interest, but the information contained in them has not been organized together or amalgamated.

PROCEDURES FOR STATEMENT SYNTHESIS

As stated at the outset of this chapter, statement synthesis involves two basic logical operations: (1) moving from observations to inferences and then (2) generalizing from specific inferences to more abstract ones. Two broad classes of methods exist for moving from observations to inferences: (1) qualitative methods and (2) quantitative methods. Generalizing from specific inferences to more general ones, the second operation, is facilitated by a process we have termed (3) literary methods. In actual statement development, a theorist may of course move back and forth between these logical operations.

Because of the complex and voluminous information about qualitative and quantitative methods, a comprehensive exposition of each is beyond the scope of this chapter. Instead we focus on strategic aspects of these two methods and must necessarily be selective in our presentation of them. Readers needing more in-depth information about qualitative methods are referred to methods texts devoted exclusively to this topic (e.g., Miles & Huberman, 1984; Leininger, 1985). Similarly, readers needing more information about quantitative methods will find standard research textbooks available on this topic (e.g., Kerlinger, 1986; Polit & Hungler, 1982). Keeping these limitations in mind, we present a treatment of qualitative, quantitative, and literary methods as they relate strategically to developing statements about a phenomenon of interest.

Qualitative methods do not use quantitative measurement. Typically, a flexible or modifiable approach is utilized in data collection. This permits the theorist to select observations related to the emerging picture of a phenomenon. Qualitative methods typically rely on interview (listening and questioning) and observation (watching) as sources of data. Field research will be presented here as an example of qualitative methods.

Quantitative methods involve measurement of variables on numerical scales. Quantitative methods may be applied to both experimental and nonexperimental (*ex post facto* or correlational) designs. In addition, quantitative methods may be further subdivided into those that focus on single subjects and those that deal with groups of subjects. Thus, four categories of quantitative designs result: single-subject experimental, single-subject nonexperimental, group experimental, and group nonexperimental. Each of these will be presented below briefly followed by further development of the use of group nonexperimental designs in statement synthesis.

Finally, literary methods are aimed at organizing extant research information on a topic of interest. Sources of evidence in literary methods rely heavily on library and printed materials. Literary methods involve sifting through available information and putting that information into more compact and general form. An example of this method will be applied to the area of disengagement in the elderly.

Qualitative Methods

Field research is probably the most widely used qualitative method of theory construction used in nursing. One especially popular version of field research, the grounded theory method (Glaser & Strauss, 1967; Glaser, 1978), has been used by nurses to study, for example, patients who underwent mastectomies (Quint, 1967a; 1967b), step-parent families (Stern, 1980), and families across life-cycle stages (Knafl & Grace, 1978). In a related field, medicine, the field method was used to study student culture in medical school (Becker et al., 1961).

A basic assumption of the field method is that the theorist can gain a better understanding of a phenomenon by beginning with an open mind and avoiding preconceived ideas about ways of classifying and interrelating data. While a theorist may begin with some general ideas about a phenomenon, these are abandoned as soon as categories more relevant to the phenomenon are defined by the theorist. The theorist moves back and forth between data collection and data analysis in order to validate emerging ideas and refine concepts and relationships as new data are collected. The field method allows a theorist to develop statements relevant to a phenomenon through using direct observation of the phenomenon as the starting point for concept and statement formation (Glaser & Strauss, 1967; Schatzman & Strauss, 1973; Glaser, 1978; Quint, 1967a). Data are coded into categories and categories are interrelated as an ongoing part of the field design. A theorist may make observations, code them, make interpretive notes or memos about coded observations, and then make further observations to refine or clarify an emerging idea. The flow of research activities in field designs is thus quite different from the compartmentalized stages of data collection, data analysis, and data interpretation in quantitative methods.

While proponents of field research methods readily acknowledge its strengths, its shortcomings must also be addressed here. Using field research methods for concept and statement construction assumes a large measure of ingenuity and intellectual integrity on the part of the theorist. Relevant concepts and relationships do not pop up in front of the theorist like mushrooms after a spring rain. The theorist's creative ability to construct general concepts and relational statements must be recognized as a crucial part of successful field research. Further, the use of perhaps hastily written field notes, selective attention to data, and errors in memory allow distortions to enter into the field research process. The theorist may, thus, inadvertantly misrepresent a phenomenon. Proponents of field methods generally argue that the empirical validity achieved by field methods offsets these shortcomings. They further argue that with careful attention and training these shortcomings of the method can be reduced substantially.

Stern (1980) has written an especially lucid account of the grounded theory method of field research. Her work with stepfather families will be used to illustrate the phases of a field method.

Stern (1980) began her study by noting that the process by which a stepfather was integrated into an existing family had not been studied before.

> . . . I had no basis on which to test existing theory, nor could I utilize identified existing variables, because none were identified. In other words, it was first necessary to find out what was going on in these families (p. 20).

During the collection of empirical data, phase one, Stern conducted intensive interviews with 30 stepfather families from a variety of social classes and ethnic groups. Data collected by observation and interviews were coded according to their main substance, and similarly coded data were then clustered together in categories. Two categories that Stern developed, for example, focused on rules in the family and enforcement techniques.

At the second phase, concept formation, a conceptual framework was developed with an eye to representing the phenomenon from the subjects' point of view. In attempting to understand how families integrate a stepfather into the existing mother-child system, Stern selected the discipline of children in the family as the framework. This framework was selected because of the emotional responses that the topic of discipline produced when discussed with families.

During the third phase, concept development, several steps occurred. Categories were linked together to define key variables. Thus, Stern combined the categories of teaching, accepting, and copying into a larger umbrella category of affiliating actions. Common to affiliating actions was bringing the stepfather and child closer together. Emerging ideas necessitated further review of literature at this point. Attention also turned to relationships between categories. In Stern's study she asked, ". . . under what conditions do the variables discipline and integration co-exist?" (p. 22). Data were selectively sampled to clarify the relationship of these variables. Stern found that discipline and integration only occurred together when affiliating actions were also present. This demonstrates statement synthesis. To further consolidate thinking, a core variable was proposed. Core variables pull together key ideas about a phenomenon. Stern proposed "integrative discipline" as the core variable explaining integration with stepfather families around the issue of discipline of children.

In the fourth phase, concept modification and integration, the emerging ideas were further integrated and delimited. Data were coded in terms of theoretical ideas. Memos or interpretive notes were made as data were coded to aid in systematizing the findings of the study. Memos were then reorganized in a manner that facilitated the fifth phase, production of the research report. In this final phase, theoretical outcomes of the study were presented substantiated by examples from the field data.

In summary, field research offers a flexible yet sensitive means of constructing statements about an empirical phenomenon. While the method of field research might also be applied to concept synthesis and theory synthesis, we believe the approach makes its greatest contribution at the level of statement synthesis. The field method permits categories and relationships among these to be constructed from direct and thoughtful interaction of the theorist and the social phenomenon being studied.

Quantitative Methods

Earlier in this chapter, four types of quantitative research designs were identified: single-subject experimental, single-subject nonexperimental, group experimental, and group nonexperimental. Each of these designs for quantitative research involves the collection and analysis of numerical data. The analysis of data typically is facilitated by statistical calculations such as means, standard deviations, percentages, correlation coefficients, and t test and F ratio values. Each of these designs contains some special advantages and limitations for the construction of statements about phenomena. To clarify these, each design will be described briefly, and then the group nonexperimental design will be presented to illustrate its use in statistically based statement synthesis.

In each of these four designs, interpreting statistical data presumes that the measurement procedures used are reliable (Anastasi, 1982; Cronbach, 1984; Nunnally, 1978). Validity of measures, particularly construct validity, may be less clear, however, given the reciprocal relationship between theory development and establishment of construct validity (Cronbach & Meehl, 1967). While it is beyond the scope of this chapter to deal with psychometric concepts such as reliability and validity as these affect the interpretation of statistical data, we must acknowledge the presence of these issues to provide a complete and accurate picture of quantitative methods applied to theory construction.

Single-Subject Designs. By single-subject designs we mean several things: (1) the careful analysis of data collected from only one individual, or (2) the analysis of data from individual subjects in the context of a group design. Both experimental (Baltes et al., 1977a; Barlow & Hersen, 1973, 1984) and nonexperimental single-subject designs permit a theorist to identify relationships between variables for individual persons. Single-subject designs prevent the masking of individual patterns of relationships that can occur when data from many subjects are pooled together. For example, in Table 7.1 and

TABLE 7.1. INDIVIDUAL AND MEAN ANXIETY LEVELS FOR PATIENTS PRIOR TO EXPLORATORY SURGERY (FICTITIOUS DATA)

Patient I.D.	Before Hospitalization	After Admission	After Preoperative Education
Patient A	50	20	20
Patient B	30	40	60
Patient C	30	50	30
Patient D	30	50	30
Group Mean	35	40	35

Figure 7.1 fictitious data on four patients about to have exploratory surgery are presented. Examining the group means for anxiety before hospitalization, after admission, and then after preoperative education gives misleading information about individual patients.

The group means suggest that patients experience an increase in anxiety after admission, but that preoperative education is successful in reducing anxiety to preadmission levels. Now looking at individual patterns, hospital admission appeared to be a relief to Patient A and reduced his anxiety level to well below preadmission levels. For Patient B, admission did raise his anxiety level somewhat, but worse yet, the preoperative education backfired and raised his level of anxiety still higher. Only Patients C and D had individual patterns that generally conformed to those of the group mean. At the beginning stages of theory building, single-subject designs such as the example given here can be an economical way of determining preliminary patterns of relationship between variables as well as suggesting whether deviations exist as individuals are compared with group patterns.

Experimental single-subject designs have been used to document the effects of nursing interventions in diverse situations: self-feeding in an elderly woman (Baltes & Zerbe, 1976) and failure to thrive in a child with Down's syndrome (Durand, 1975). Baltes and Zerbe reported use of a reinforcement program to initiate and maintain self-feeding behavior in an elderly woman confined to a nursing home. Base line frequencies of self-feeding behaviors were measured

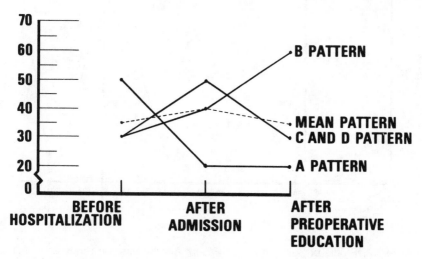

Figure 7.1. Individual and Mean Anxiety Levels for Patients Prior to Exploratory Surgery (Fictitious Data)

before the reinforcement treatment began. During and after the treatment (intervention) phase, frequency of self-feeding behaviors was measured each day. As Figure 7.2 shows, the frequency of self-feeding behaviors in the elderly subject was dependent upon the differing reinforcements presented during the base line and treatment phases of the research. From the data, Baltes and Zerbe concluded: "nonfeeding is an 'operant' in old age which can be changed into self-feeding, depending on environmental contingencies" (p. 26).

As shown in the two examples above, examining the impact of an intervention on a small number of individuals can be helpful in clarifying the varied ways that variables may be interrelated and identifying types of persons for whom the intervention may be unsuitable. Single-subject experimental designs are, of course, limited in external validity or generalizability. Such designs may, however, be the birthplace of ideas later refined and tested in group designs.

In a nonexperimental context, examining data on a single-subject basis and comparing this with group patterns may be helpful

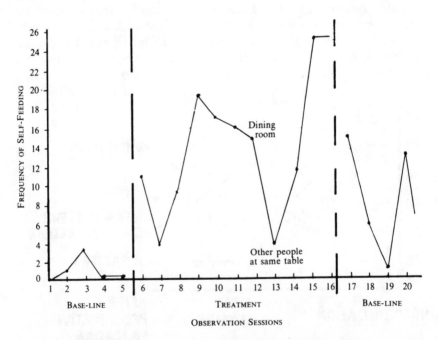

Figure 7.2. Profile of Self-Feeding of Patient A in 20-Session Study. *From Baltes MM, Zerbe MB: Reestablishing self-feeding in a nursing home resident. Nurs Res 25:26, 1976.*

in identifying naturally occurring deviant patterns that are clinically important. Thoman (1980) has presented an interesting example of this approach. In studying the sleep-awake patterns of infants, she observed the percent of awake time infants spend during 7-hr observations made at 2, 3, 4, and 5 weeks of age. As Figure 7.3 shows, one infant, "S," demonstrated markedly higher percentages of awake time (eyes open and alert), particularly at the 5-week period, in contrast to other infants. This pattern was later linked to neurological impairment in that infant. Careful observations, recordings, and comparison of sleep-awake patterns of this infant allowed Thoman to formulate the relationship between neurological impairment in midinfancy and early sleep-awake patterns. Thoman's quantitative approach permitted a relationship to be identified that might have gone unnoticed if the data had been recorded only on a qualitative basis.

Individual-subject designs are mentioned here both because they

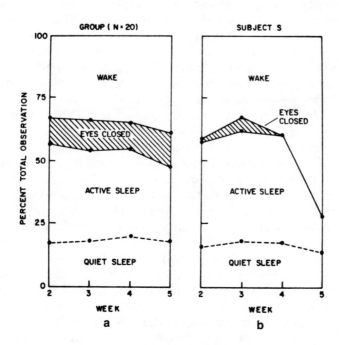

Figure 7.3. Distribution of States During 7-Hr Observation at 2, 3, 4, and 5 Weeks of Age. **(a)** Mean Values for Group of Normal Infants; **(b)** Individual Values for Subject S. *From Thoman EB: Infant development viewed in the mother-infant relationship. In (EJ Quilligan, N Kretchmer, eds.), Fetal and Maternal Medicine, New York: Wiley, 1980, 257.*

are an often overlooked approach to theory development in nursing and because they offer economy. The time and resources required for a single-subject design are especially appealing where time and resources are precious.

Group Designs. As we pointed out earlier, group designs may be either experimental or nonexperimental. In a group experimental design, a "treatment" or experimental condition is applied to a group of subjects. Observations or measurements are then taken to determine the impact of the experimental condition on some outcome variable. To aid the interpretation of a group experimental design, a control group may be included so that the effects of the experimental condition on subjects may be contrasted with the effects of the control condition. If only an experimental group of subjects is feasible, subjects may be tested both before and after the experimental condition is applied so that a meaningful point of contrast exists for the outcome variable.

A variety of more elaborate group experimental designs can be built from these two basic experimental models. These designs are well documented in research design and statistics texts (e.g., Kerlinger, 1986; Shelley, 1984), so they will not be presented here. Rather we wish to point out that the group experimental design, while widely used as a hypothesis testing method, may also be useful in hypothesis-generating research. One of the primary drawbacks of the use of the method in a discovery context is its lack of economy in contrast to single-subject designs. Where the sample drawn for exploratory work is in line with those in the larger population, however, group experimental designs offer greater external validity or generalizability of synthesized conclusions.

The final quantitative method to be considered here is the group nonexperimental design. Such designs typically use correlation or regression techniques to statistically interrelate variables. Data may be cross-sectional (collected at one time frame) or longitudinal (collected over several time frames). While we will not discuss the variety of test statistics that may be used in nonexperimental (also called correlational or *ex post facto*) designs, we will discuss general strategies for the analysis and interpretation of nonexperimental data. Associated statistical and design issues are well treated in available research texts (e.g., Achenbach, 1978; Baltes et al., 1977b; Polit & Hungler, 1982).

Probably the greatest problem that group nonexperimental designs pose for a theorist is the risk of becoming buried in a sea of statistical information. The "shotgun" approach often used in nonexperimental designs can result in every variable being related to every other variable in the study. In a study of ten variables (for example, social class, age, sex, number of drugs, number of hospital admissions, and so on), if each of these is correlated with every other variable, a total of 45 correlation coefficients will be generated. In a study of 100 variables, 4950 variable relationships are possible. Immediately it becomes clear that strategies are needed to eliminate unnecessary statistical analyses and to organize those that are done into meaningful units of information. This is one of the most difficult tasks that faces a theorist using quantitative nonexperimental evidence for statement synthesis.

To organize the process of data analysis and interpretation, we recommend several guidelines.

1. Locate the most focal variables, those of greatest interest to you. Some variables are of interest for their own sake, for example, levels of adjustment or well-being before or after illness. Other variables are of interest primarily only in so far as they may influence focal variables.

2. Examine the statistical indicators of central tendency and variability on the focal variables (Jacobsen, 1981). If these variables are measured over several occasions, become familiar with changes that may occur in them.

3. Examine related literature for variables that have been found to covary with these focal variables.

4. Determine if your focal variables are related as expected to these variables identified in the literature.

5. Reduce variables that seem to have a common orientation by such procedures as factor analysis (Tabachnick & Fidell, 1983, pp. 372–445) if possible. Social background variables can often be made more compact by this approach.

6. Follow up hunches that you may have about new variables in your data set that you suspect may be related to the focal variables.

7. Look for "surprises" in the data analysis results. These may be unanticipated relationships or unanticipated lack of relationships. Hypothesize about why these surprises may have occurred. Check out your hypotheses to the extent possible with your available data. These hypotheses, while moving beyond statement synthesis itself, may be helpful for later theory synthesis.

8. While you may have started out atheoretically (without any theory in mind to be proven), you may find during the data analysis and interpretation phase that the results obtained are consistent with available theories. These theories may in turn suggest new or previously unexplored areas for further analysis of the data.

9. Discuss results obtained with colleagues knowledgeable in the

area as well as with clinicians who know the area under study from a case by case perspective.

The suggestions above are guidelines and not rules for data analysis. Keeping a log of what was done and why may also be helpful in directing the analysis of data in new but organized directions. Review the log frequently. Writing summaries of the results of completed data analyses may also be a useful reference point. Review these summaries, discuss them with colleagues, and compare them with results of published research. Occasionally, reading about research that is unrelated but similar in design can be helpful in organizing and guiding the data analysis in new and meaningful directions.

We will present a small segment of data from a group nonexperimental study that one of us completed. We will demonstrate the use of quantitative data in statement synthesis. (Data were gathered with support from grant number NU 00677. Division of Nursing, U.S. Public Health Service, 1978–1981.) In one part of the study, attitudes and beliefs of new mothers were investigated. Because the literature suggested that maternal parity and infant sex might influence attitudes and beliefs, data were analyzed separately according to parity (primiparas and multiparas) and infant sex (male and female) subgroups. While this division reduced the number of subjects within groups, it provided a sharper picture of attitudes or belief patterns among new mothers. Table 7.2 presents the correlations between three attitudes and beliefs measured at the beginning and at the end of the neonatal period. The correlations are presented for each of the four subgroups of new mothers. The correlation of mothers' attitudes toward themselves as mothers are quite high for all four subgroups ($r = 0.62$–0.77). Thus, one might claim that mothers' attitudes toward themselves as mothers do not undergo major changes during the neonatal period, that is, overall attitude toward oneself as mother was a relatively stable phenomenon across time regardless of parity or sex of infant. For beliefs about one's infant, however, this is not true. Beliefs about one's baby were significantly correlated across the neonatal period for primiparous mothers ($r = 0.35$ to 0.41), but not for multiparas ($r = -0.06$ to -0.12). Thus, beliefs about one's baby are somewhat stable for first-time mothers; for mothers having other than a first baby, beliefs at the end of the neonatal period are unrelated to initial beliefs.

This latter finding was indeed surprising. One might have expected that inexperienced mothers would have unrealistic beliefs about infants so that they would be the group most likely to change their beliefs over the course of the neonatal period. What we hypoth-

TABLE 7.2. CORRELATION BETWEEN NEW MOTHERS' ATTITUDES/BELIEFS AT THE BEGINNING AND END OF THE NEONATAL PERIOD[a]

Maternal Parity/ Infant Sex	Attitude/Belief		
	Beliefs About Baby	Attitude Toward Baby	Attitude Toward Self as Mother
Primiparous/Female	0.35[b] (28)	0.44[c] (31)	0.62[d] (31)
Primiparous/Male	0.41[c] (42)	0.44[c] (43)	0.66[d] (43)
Multiparous/Female	−0.06 (51)	0.69[d] (51)	0.67[d] (51)
Multiparous/Male	−0.12 (35)	0.23 (38)	0.77[d] (38)

[a]Numbers of subjects are in parentheses. These may vary within groups because of some missing data.
[b] $= p < .05$.
[c] $= p < .01$.
[d] $= p < .001$.

esized happened is this. First-time mothers, because of their inexperience with infants, "stereotype" them. Thus, when the infant's early behavior is different from expectations, these behaviors are ignored and the stereotype is maintained. Mothers who have already had at least one child have learned over time that babies are very individual as they compared their earlier babies' growth and behavior with other babies. Thus, "repeat" mothers did not expect babies to conform to a stereotype. As a result, "repeat" mothers change their initial beliefs about their later babies more readily than first-time mothers as they come to know their individual behaviors. Explanations other than this one, of course, may also be given for the surprising results reported here.

Now look at the column in Table 7.2 labeled "Attitude Toward Baby." Make a statement about how consistent across time mothers' attitudes toward their babies were for the four groups. Try to construct a reason that would explain the statement you made.

In constructing your statement, you should have noted that mothers' attitudes toward their babies were significantly related across the neonatal period for all four groups of mothers ($r = 0.44$– 0.69) except for multiparous mothers of male infants ($r = 0.23$). Several hypotheses explaining this finding may be offered. We hypothesize that mothers of first borns stereotype their babies so that their attitudes remain somewhat consistent over time regardless of their infant's sex. Let us assume, however, that male infants as a group are more unpredictable or variable than females in the first weeks of life. If we further assume that multiparous mothers are more aware of individuality of infants, we might then expect that multiparous mothers of male infants might change their attitudes more than other mothers in response to the variability of their babies. Your reasons may be as plausible as the ones offered here. Given the limited information we have provided here, there is no single best explanation. Examining the available data would help to evaluate the plausibility of the explanation we have given here. For example, the data might be examined to determine if male infants were indeed more variable than females in the neonatal period.

While we have given a number of guidelines for the analysis and interpretation of quantitative nonexperimental data, we have not stated exact procedures for the application of this method. We have avoided stating procedures because we did not want to mislead readers into believing that statement synthesis is a mechanical process of inspecting data and then simply formulating statements from the data. A key strategic aspect of statistically based statement synthesis is in the organization of the data analysis. We have tried to emphasize this aspect, being assured that research methods texts amply cover procedural aspects of quantitative nonexperimental research (Polit & Hungler, 1982; Kidder & Judd, 1986; Baltes et al., 1977b). We believe the information on strategic aspects of quantitative methods in a discovery context presented here is unaddressed in conventional research texts.

Implicit in our treatment of quantitative methods has been a threefold process: (1) approach data analysis in inventive yet organized ways, (2) carefully describe results via systematic formulation of statements, and (3) where possible, link statements derived from data with existing theories or hypothesized explanations. While the third phase moves beyond statement synthesis itself, it is meaningful to include it here in order to set the stage for other theoretical activities such as theory synthesis and theory testing.

Quantitative methods in general offer theorists the advantage of access to explicit numerical data about a phenomenon. While numbers may lack the flavor of reality, they can aid relationship identification in ways the naked eye may miss. Relationships are in the end an abstraction about reality, not reality itself. Quantitative methods can facilitate the abstraction process in that their application to reality forces a theorist to think about reality in conceptual and quantitative dimensions. Temperature is not simply "hot" or "cold" but a specific reading on a temperature gauge. Similarly, social and psychological concepts such as "liking" may be translated into scores on scales for voice tone, touching behaviors, and visual contact. Quantitative methods require the continuing and thoughtful attention of the theorist in the data analytic and interpretive processes, however, lest the theorist become lost in an array of numbers.

Literary Methods

Literary methods of statement synthesis start out with statements derived from extant research. In contrast to statement analysis, literary methods of statement synthesis utilize only those statements in scientific literature that are derived or supported by empirical evidence. Relationships that are conjectural on a theorist's part or that are not founded on research findings are not included. This criterion for statement inclusion does not necessarily mean that conjectures or unsupported statements are not useful in theory construction. Rather the criterion reflects the orientation of synthesis strategies: to begin theoretical work from empirical evidence. Conjectural or unsupported statements fail to meet this criterion. Conjectural statements may be useful, however, in other types of strategies, such as statement analysis or statement derivation.

The following statement was empirically supported in Henthorn's (1979) study of disengagement and reinforcement in the elderly:

> . . . the greater the degree of disengagement [reported by the elderly], the lower the level of reinforcement [of role behaviors by others] and the anticipated reinforcement [of role behaviors by others] (p. 5).

Often statements such as the example above need to be rewritten to clarify their meaning. In this example, the statement in fact describes two sets of relationships, which may be restated as follows:

> the greater the degree of disengagement reported by the elderly, the lower the level of reinforcement of role behaviors by others,

and

> the greater the degree of disengagement reported by the elderly, the lower the anticipated reinforcement of role behaviors by others.

There are several essentially equivalent forms in which relational statements such as these above may be written. Examples of these forms follow.

> The greater the X, the greater the Y.
> As X increases (or decreases), Y increases (or decreases).
> X and Y covary.
> X is positively (or negatively) related to Y.

The form in which these statements are written is ambiguous. Left open are several questions:

1. Is the relationship between X and Y reversible, that is, if an increase in X is related to an increase in Y, is an increase in Y also related to an increase in X?
2. Is the relationship between the two variables X and Y causal or noncausal (simply associative)?

These questions can only be answered if the design of the research from which the statement was derived was aimed at disentangling these issues. Otherwise, the theorist must simply recognize the ambiguity and await further research that can clarify the answers to the reversibility and causality questions.

Typically, experimental approaches help clarify questions left ambiguous by correlational or nonexperimental designs. There are correlational techniques, for example, cross-lagged panel correlations, which can shed some light on questions about directions of influence between variables (Baltes et al., 1977b). Where answers to questions about causality and reversibility can be answered, the form in which statements may be written is more precise. For example,

> Only if there is an increase in X, will there be an increase in Y, but the reverse is not true (nonreversible or unidirectional causality),

or

> Only if there is an increase in X, will there be an increase in Y, and vice versa (reversibility or bidirectional causality).

Literary statement synthesis occurs through either of two techniques: (1) by making the meanings of the concepts included in a statement more general, or (2) by expanding the boundaries (scope of phenomena covered) to include a wider variety of situations. The first of these may be done by merging less general concepts into one more abstract, general concept. The latter is done by reformulating the boundaries of a statement to increase the populations and situations to which it applies; for example, extending statements about small group interaction patterns to all groups regardless of size. We will apply both of these techniques of literary synthesis. Our first revised statement taken from Henthorn will be the starting point:

> The greater the degree of disengagement reported by the elderly, the lower the level of reinforcement of role behaviors by others.

Now let us take a statement from Osofsky and Danzger's research on early mother-infant interaction (1974). They noted that:

> the attentive mother tends to have a responsive baby and vice versa (p. 124).

We will attempt to synthesize the findings of Henthorn's and Osofsky and Danzger's studies by first developing a broader concept from the concepts "degree of disengagement" and "attentive mother." Common to these two concepts is a more general concept: "amount of social interactive behaviors an individual emits." For the concepts "level of reinforcement of role behaviors by others" and "responsive baby," a commonality exists in the higher-order concept "social reinforcement that accompanies social interactive behaviors." We further broaden the situational scope of our statement by shifting the boundaries from the elderly or mothers and infants to an individual in social interaction with others. Thus, a synthesized statement drawn from Henthorn's and Osofsky and Danzger's studies may be made.

> The amount of social interactive behaviors an individual emits is directly related to the amount of social reinforcement received from others.

Finally, because we were unclear about the reversibility of Henthorn's statement, we chose a conservative interpretation of it and wrote the synthesized statement as nonreversible.

In the example of social interaction and reinforcement we have tried to show how a general statement may be synthesized from two statements that initially appear dissimilar. This was done to help the reader grasp the basic, and sometimes surprising, ways in which research outcomes can be pulled together into synthesized statements. Formulating a statement that generalizes to new and broader boundaries, of course, requires that additional data be sought to substantiate the new generalization. Nonetheless, an important move in theory construction may have been made as further evidence is being awaited.

Literary methods of statement synthesis may be given a still further level of scrutiny. Where a series of statements has been synthesized from research literature on a phenomenon, statements may be ranked or classified according to the level of empirical support available to substantiate them (see, e.g., Sears, 1972, pp. 23–25). Statements that have supporting evidence collected in multiple studies using diverse populations would be ranked more highly than those with a more limited base of evidence. Particularly where research findings are used as a basis for public policy formation or for application to practice, clear determination of the extent of support for synthesized statements is important.

Statement synthesis from literary sources, while time consuming, involves minimal cost and resources compared to other statement synthesis methods. Access to adequate library facilities is crucial to this method. Literary approaches to statement synthesis are especially useful in that statements generated are not limited to the findings of any one study. Access to findings of multiple studies on a topic of interest offers a richer data base than any single study. Literary approaches will be only partly satisfactory, however, where the published research on a topic is limited in amount and quality.

ADVANTAGES AND LIMITATIONS

Because methods of statement synthesis are so varied, we will speak to advantages and limitations in only the most general terms here. An evaluation of the advantages and limitations of statement synthesis methods as a group hinges on philosophical assumptions that are discussed below.

Statement synthesis as a method assumes that confrontation with reality is a useful and productive means of constructing theory. It assumes that without the aid of a clear guiding theory a theorist can detect the dimensions of a phenomenon that are the most scientifically useful. In describing such atheoretical approaches to theory construction as "research-then-theory," Reynolds (1971) noted that they assume there are real patterns that exist in nature. These patterns are then discovered by researchers using empirical methods. In this viewpoint, "research" is akin to "search." Reynolds further notes that the assumptions made about how scientific knowledge relates to the real world are philosophical and thus not amenable to resolution by scientific methods. We thus also must leave our readers to decide for themselves, using philosophical methods, if they find the assumptions of synthetic methods tenable. This issue goes beyond the scope of this book. We hope that readers will find these philosophical issues as intriguing as the more procedural ones treated in this book.

UTILIZING THE RESULTS OF STATEMENT SYNTHESIS

Formulating statements about nursing phenomena from observations (both qualitatively and quantitatively recorded) and from published research is the aim of statement synthesis. Utilizing the results of this strategy leads directly into the larger knowledge-generating process. Thus, this strategy forms the substance of reviewing research literature as a preamble to a study. It also is employed in reaching study conclusions and transmitting those conclusions through the educational process. In many respects, statement synthesis is the same thing as the research process and the educational process. If the researcher and teacher are committed to carefully grounding their work on scientific observation, then statement synthesis is not a product used but rather a process at the heart of what each does.

These general comments aside, statements carefully formulated from research and observation are needed particularly in undergraduate nursing education. While "concept" teaching may provide the foci of nursing content, only when concepts are linked within statements do explanations and predictions become possible. The latter form the base for making logical inferences in relating content to practice. Thus, synthesized statements may be used to enrich the content of nursing instruction.

SUMMARY

Statement synthesis is an empirically based strategy for constructing statements that specify the manner in which two or more concepts are interrelated. The strategy encompasses a number of diverse approaches to developing theory. Specific methods range from field research to an assortment of quantitative approaches to library search and amalgamation.

The field research, a qualitative method, places a heavy burden on theorists to be perceptive of processes that underlie the events they confront in the field. Quantitative approaches begin with identifying numerical ways of observing reality. These are then analyzed with the aid of statistical methods to sharpen the patterns inherent in data. Literary methods aim at pulling together general statements of relationships from available research. Despite the diversity of these methods, they share in common a dependence on evidence for formulating scientific statements and a common philosophical assumption about how scientific knowledge reflects reality.

PRACTICE EXERCISES

Table 7.3 is a continuation of the study of new mothers' beliefs and attitudes reported earlier in this chapter. The information in the table addresses the relationship of attitudes toward the baby and attitudes toward oneself as mother as each of these relate to beliefs about the baby. The correlations between these measures were based on data collected at the end of the neonatal period. As before, the correlations are reported separately by parity or sex groups.

Inspect the information in Table 7.3 carefully. Formulate one or more statements about how sex or parity groups are similar or differ-

TABLE 7.3. CORRELATION BETWEEN NEW
MOTHERS' ATTITUDES AND BELIEFS AT THE END
OF THE NEONATAL PERIOD[a]

| | Correlation Among Attitudes Beliefs[b] | |
Maternal Parity/ Infant Sex/	Beliefs about Baby and Attitude Toward Baby	Beliefs about Baby and Attitude Toward Self as Mother
Primiparous/Female	−0.59[c] (28)	−0.67[c] (28)
Primiparous/Male	−0.50[c] (43)	−0.26 (43)
Multiparous/Female	−0.39[d] (49)	0.14 (49)
Multiparous/Male	−0.28 (34)	−0.13 (34)

[a]Number of subjects are in parentheses.
[b]The negative sign (−0.00) on the correlations is an artifact of the opposite
direction in which the attitude and belief scales are scored; for this exercise
the negative sign on the correlations may be ignored and the correlations
treated essentially as positive relations between variables.
[c] $= p < .001$.
[d] $= p < .01$.

ent in terms of relationships reported. Formulate an explanation for
the results as you stated them.

From an inspection of the data you should have noted that for all
mothers, except multiparous mothers of males, beliefs about one's
baby and attitude toward one's baby were significantly correlated.
However, beliefs about one's baby and attitude toward oneself as
mother were uncorrelated within all groups except primiparous
mothers of girls.

Since we have earlier offered explanations for the unique features of the relationship of a multiparous mother and her male infant, we will not repeat those here. That line of reasoning would help
to explain the pattern of correlations between beliefs about the baby
and attitude toward baby.

For the correlation patterns of parity or sex groups for the variables beliefs about baby and attitude toward self as mother, we hypothesize the following. Mothers construct "world views" of
themselves and how they relate to their infants. The mothers' attitude toward themselves may either be integrated with their beliefs
about their babies or distinct from them. Where mothers are confi-
dent in themselves, their views of themselves will be distinct or
separate from how they see their infants. Also, where mothers hold
beliefs about their babies that are many times proven wrong, they
will also tend to separate their beliefs about their babies from their
attitude toward themselves. Multiparous mothers are likely to view
their babies separately from themselves because of their confidence

in themselves as successful mothers in the past. For different reasons, such as unpredictable behavior of the male infant, primiparous mothers of males will also separate their beliefs about their infants from their attitude toward themselves as mothers. Only first-time mothers of females are able to integrate their attitude toward themselves with their beliefs about their infants.

Again as before, your explanation may be as plausible as the one offered here. What is most important, however, is that you should now be able to look at data, describe it, and hypothesize about reasons behind it.

PRETEST ON STATISTICS

1. Overall, the best predictor of any individual's score on a test is the
   A. Variance
   B. Standard deviation
   C. Correlation
   D. Mean
2. Changing an individual's raw scores on several tests into percentages has what effect?
   A. Splits an individual score into quartiles
   B. Locks an individual's scores into a common unit
   C. Establishes the group mean
   D. Results in the calculation of the group variance
3. The χ^2 statistic is designed to analyze data that are
   A. Categorical (noncontinuous)
   B. Ordinal (rank-ordered)
   C. Interval (equal interval)
   D. Ratio (true zero point)
4. A correlation coefficient reflects the
   A. Average deviation from the mean
   B. Difference between two means
   C. Relationship between two variables
   D. Most frequently occurring score in a score distribution
5. A t test and analysis of variance (ANOVA) are similar in that both
   A. Apply to categorical data
   B. Test the differences between means
   C. Test the relationship between variables
   D. May be used to compute the variance
6. Nurse A collected information on which patients kept or broke their clinic appointments during one month. Further, Nurse A classified all these patients as "teenagers" or "nonteenagers" in order to determine if teenagers had special problems in keeping

appointments. To analyze Nurse A's data, the most appropriate statistic is which of the following?

A. Measure of central tendency

B. χ^2

C. Correlated t test

D. Analysis of variance

7. In analyzing some other data about clinic patients, Nurse A calculated a correlation coefficient of $+2.19$. The size of the correlation indicates

A. A strong relationship

B. A large difference

C. A significant finding

D. An error in calculation

8. The director of the clinic told Nurse A that evidence was needed to show the effectiveness of the patient education done in the clinic. Nurse A decided to compare hypertensive patients' systolic blood pressures before and after the patient education program one year ago. To do this, Nurse A should use which test statistic?

A. A measure of deviation from the mean

B. χ^2

C. Correlation

D. Analysis of variance

Answers: 1. D; 2. B; 3. A; 4. C; 5. B; 6. B; 7. D; 8. D

REFERENCES

Achenbach TM: Research in Developmental Psychology: Concepts, Strategies, Methods. New York: Free Press, 1978.

Anastasi A: Psychological Testing. 5th ed. New York: Collier, 1982.

Baltes MM, Zerbe MB: Reestablishing self-feeding in a nursing home resident. Nurs Res 25: 24–26, 1976.

Baltes PB, Reese HW, Nesselroade JR: Chapter 23. Developmental research on learning: Single-subject designs. In Life-Span Developmental Psychology: Introduction to Research Methods. Monterey, Calif.: Brooks/Cole, 1977a.

Baltes PB, Reese HW, Nesselroade JR: Life-Span Developmental Psychology: Introduction to Research Methods. Monterey, Calif.: Brooks/Cole, 1977b.

Barlow DH, Hersen M: Single-case experimental designs. Arch Gen Psychiatr 29: 319–325, 1973.

Barlow DH, Hersen M: Single-Case Experimental Designs. 2d ed. New York: Pergamon, 1984.

Becker HS, Geer B, Hughes EC, Strauss ASL: Boys in White. Chicago: Univ. of Chicago, 1961.

Cronbach LJ: Essentials of Psychological Testing. 4th ed. New York: Harper & Row, 1984.

Cronbach LJ, Meehl PE: Construct validity in psychological tests. In (DN Jackson & S Messick, eds.), Problems in Human Assessment. New York: McGraw-Hill, 1967.

Durand B: Failure to thrive in a child with Down's syndrome. Nurs Res 24: 272–286, 1975.

Glaser BG: Theoretical Sensitivity. Mill Valley, Calif.: Sociology Press, 1978.

Glaser BG, Strauss AL: The Discovery of Grounded Theory: Strategies for Qualitative Research. Chicago: Aldine, 1967.

Henthorn BS: Disengagement and reinforcement in the elderly. Res Nurs Health 2: 1–8, 1979.

Jacobsen BS: Know thy data. Nurs Res 30: 254–255, 1981.

Kerlinger FN: Foundations of Behavioral Research. 3rd ed. New York: Holt, Rinehart & Winston, 1986.

Kidder L, Judd CM: Research Methods in Social Relations. 5th ed. New York: Holt, Rinehart & Winston, 1986.

Knafl KA, Grace HK (eds.): Families Across the Life Cycle. Boston: Little, Brown, 1978.

Leininger M: Qualitative Research Methods in Nursing. New York: Grune & Stratton, 1985.

Miles MB, Huberman AM: Qualitative Data Analysis. Beverly Hills: Sage, 1984.

Nunnally JC: Psychometric Theory. 2d ed. New York: McGraw-Hill, 1978.

Osofsky JD, Danzger B: Relationships between neonatal characteristics and mother-infant interaction. Devel Psychol 10: 124–130, 1974.

Polit DF, Hungler BP: Nursing Research: Principles and Methods. 2d ed. Philadelphia: Lippincott, 1982.

Quint JC: The case for theories generated from empirical data. Nurs Res 16: 109–114, 1967a.

Quint JC: The Nurse and the Dying Patient. New York: Macmillan, 1967b.

Reynolds PD: A Primer in Theory Construction. Indianapolis: Bobbs-Merrill, 1971.

Schatzman L, Strauss AL: Field Research: Strategies for a Natural Sociology. Englewood Cliffs, N. J.: Prentice-Hall, 1973.

Sears RR: Attachment, dependency, and frustration. In (JL Gerwitz, ed.), Attachment and Dependency. New York: John Wiley, 1–27, 1972.

Shelley SI: Research Methods in Nursing and Health. Boston: Little, Brown, 1984.

Stern PN: Grounded theory methodology: Its uses and processes. Image 12: 20–23, 1980.

Tabachnick BG, Fidell LS: Using Multivariate Statistics. Philadelphia: Harper & Row, 1983.

Thoman EB: Infant development viewed in the mother-infant relationship. In (EJ Quilligan & N Kretchmer, eds.), Fetal and Maternal Medicine. New York: John Wiley, 1980.

ADDITIONAL READINGS

Readings in Statistics

Guilford JP, Fruchter B: Fundamental Statistics in Psychology and Education. 6th ed. New York: McGraw-Hill, 1978.

Huck SW, Cormier WH, Bounds WG: Readings in Statistics and Research. New York: Harper & Row, 1974.
Williams F: Reasoning with Statistics. 3d ed. New York: Holt, Rinehart & Winston, 1986.
Young RK, Veldman DJ: Introductory Statistics for the Behavioral Sciences. 4th ed. New York: Holt, Rinehart & Winston, 1981.

Readings in Statement Construction

Dubin R: Theory Building. New York: The Free Press, 1978.
Hage J: Techniques and Problems of Theory Construction in Sociology. New York: John Wiley, 1972.
Mullins NC: The Art of Theory: Construction and Use. New York: Harper & Row, 1971.
Olson S: Ideas and Data: The Process and Practice of Social Research. Homewood, Ill.: Dorsey, 1976.
Pillemer DB, Light RJ: Synthesizing outcomes: How to use research evidence from many studies. Harvard Ed Rev 50: 176–195, 1980.
Reynolds PD: A Primer in Theory Construction. Indianapolis: Bobbs-Merrill, 1971.
Zetterberg HL: On Theory and Verification in Sociology. Totowa, N. J.: Bedminister Press, 1965.

8

Statement Derivation

DEFINITION AND DESCRIPTION

Statement derivation is a strategy for developing a set of statements about a phenomenon by using an analogy. A set of statements (S_1) from one field of interest (F_1) is used to derive the content or structure of a second set of statements (S_2) for a second field (F_2). Thus, a second series of statements is created that shares some common structural or content features with an existing set of statements. Despite similar structure or terminology, the two sets of statements are distinct because each refers to a separate field of interest (see Figure 8.1).

Identifying an analogy or likeness between phenomena in two different fields is the basis of statement derivation. The likeness or analogy between statements in two fields may be either substantive or formal. In a *substantive analogy* the likeness rests in the content or concepts in two fields. In a *formal analogy* it is the logical structure linking together concepts in one field that is analogous to or like a second field. On the surface, the two fields of interest do not neces-

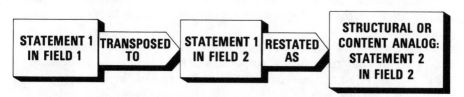

Figure 8.1. Process of Statement Derivation

sarily have to appear similar. All that is required is that there be analogous dimensions between phenomena in the two fields. For example, let us assume there is a statement in physical science that states that for any two objects in motion close to each other, there are forces that attract the objects to each other as well as forces that repel them. By analogy, we might theorize that for any two persons who are in close physical contact with each other, there are forces that attract the persons to each other as well as forces that repel them. Despite gross differences in the phenomena in the two fields, these two statements bear a structural and content similarity to each other.

The processes for deriving the content and structure of statements are crucial to understanding statement derivation. Deriving the *content* and *structure* of a new statement from an existing "parent" statement involves two logically separate derivations. While a theorist might simultaneously carry out the content and structural aspects of statement derivation, we will separate them to present each aspect more clearly.

Derivation of the content of a new statement is akin to concept derivation (see Chapter 5). What a theorist does is specify the terms or concepts to be included in a new statement and their accompanying definitions within the new field. Derivation of the structure of the new statements entails specifying the type of linkage between the newly derived concepts or terms. The linkage may be a unidirectional causal relationship, a simple positive relationship, a negative association, or a more complex algebraic relationship. (See Chapters 6 and 7 for a further discussion of the types of linkages within statements.)

Let's look at the following sample statement that will be used to derive a statement about family interaction.

> When the volume of a gas is held constant, the temperature and pressure are positively related.

Content derivation focuses on specifying family terminology to parallel the key chemical concepts or terms in this statement: gas, volume, temperature, and pressure. For example, the terms "family," "amount of interaction," "amount of hostile comments," and "amount of angry responses" might be defined as respective analogs of the chemical terminology.

In looking at the structural derivation of a new statement, content terms that refer to the properties of the phenomenon, for example, pressure, may be eliminated and replaced by simple placeholding symbols such as A, B, and C. Thus, our beginning statement may be rewritten as follows:

> When the *A* of a *B* is held constant, the *C* and *D* are positively related.

This noncontent statement presents only the skeleton or structure of relationships among our unspecified concepts or terms: *A*, *B*, *C*, and *D*. As written, the statement makes logical sense but does not have any meaning in terms of real phenomena. Until *A–D* are defined by terms having meanings in reality, the statement is not empirically interpretable. To specify meanings for *A–D*, let us substitute the terms developed earlier for family interaction.

> When the amount of interaction of a family is held constant, the amount of hostile comments and the amount of angry responses are positively related.

With this last step, the derivation of a statement about family interaction is completed. Not all cases of statement derivation need entail both content and structural derivation aspects. If a theorist has already delineated relevant concepts describing a phenomenon and only lacks a clear mode of interrelating them, only the structural aspect of statement derivation may be needed.

Parallels in the structure or content of statements across fields are based on the analogy that a theorist identifies as implicit between two fields of interest. As a result, a large measure of the success of statement derivation hinges on the theorist's insightful selection of an existing field that contains rich parallels with the theorist's field of interest. There is no set rule for selecting timely and fruitful "parent" fields from which to begin statement derivation. A theorist's "sense" or awareness of phenomena in the field of interest is certainly an important ingredient. Reading in fields that are related as well as unrelated to the theorist's interests also can establish a range of alternate fields from which to begin statement derivation. The true heuristic value of a parent field can only be determined as a theorist actually attempts to derive statements from a parent field.

PURPOSE AND USES

The purpose of statement derivation is to formulate one or more statements about a phenomenon that is currently not well understood. Statement derivation is especially suited to situations in which (1) no available data base or body of literature exists, or (2) current thinking is becoming outmoded and new perspectives are needed. Statement derivation is especially relevant where a theorist

does not wish to provide an integrated theoretical model of a phenomenon but merely wishes to clarify how several dimensions of a
phenomenon are related. For example, suppose a theorist wishes to
clarify how nurse support relates to coping with pain experienced
during intrusive diagnostic procedures. Suppose the theorist finds
literature on patient preparation before procedures but none on support during the procedure itself. Because the theorist is particularly
interested in diagnostic procedures done when little or no preparation is feasible, the focus of interest is limited to support given during procedures. Patient preparation would in this context be less
relevant and a theorist might justifiably choose to limit theorizing to
one or two statements about the phenomenon in question: nurse
support during intrusive diagnostic procedures.

In addition, suppose that the literature the theorist finds about
nurse support during diagnostic procedures is simply, "Support the
patient." Clearly, a more penetrating and innovative way of thinking
about nurse support is needed. An entire theory, however, may not be
needed. An exercise in statement derivation may be the most reasonable and rapid means of developing one or more statements about
nurse support during intrusive procedures. We will continue with the
example of nurse support in the next section.

PROCEDURES FOR STATEMENT DERIVATION

Statement derivation may be broken down into several steps. In
actual practice, a theorist may move through several steps almost
simultaneously or occasionally repeat steps to improve the final
results. The steps are, thus, guideposts rather than rigid lock-step
maneuvers in theory building. Bearing this in mind, we list the steps
in statement derivation below.

1. Become thoroughly familiar with any existing literature on one's
   topic of interest. This should involve not only reading but also
   critically evaluating the level of usefulness of statements about
   the topic of interest. This step should confirm the need to use the
   statement derivation strategy: need for a new perspective should
   be evident.
2. Search other fields for new ways of looking at the topic of interest.
   Read literature from several fields, some similar to and some
   dissimilar from the topic and field of interest. Be alert to those
   aspects of the literature that specifically express the major relational statements of each field.
3. Select the parent field to be used in the derivation process, and

carefully identify the structural and content features of the parent statements to be used in derivations. Be sure to separately consider both the structural suitability and the content suitability of statements in the parent field. Because derivation is not a mechanical process, the theorist is free to modify statements in the parent field to increase their suitability to the derivation process. Thus, statements from the parent field may be restated to enhance their clarity and to more sharply display the structure of relationships between concepts.

4. Develop new statements about the topic of interest from the content and structure of statements in the parent field. This step, simply stated, consists of restating the parent statements in terms of the subject matter of the new field, that is, the theorist's topic of interest.

5. Redefine any new concepts or terms in the derived statements to fit the specific subject matter of the topic of interest. If statement derivation is used only to provide the structure for interrelating concepts that already exist in the field of interest, much of this step may already be done. Even so, it is prudent to reassess the suitability of definitions of terms when they are placed within the structure of new statements. Adaptations in meaning may be needed.

To illustrate these steps in operation, we will continue to explore the hypothetical case of the nurse theorist interested in nurse support during painful diagnostic procedures. For this illustration let us assume that no research has been conducted to examine the specific effect of nurse support on patient coping with pain during diagnostic procedures. The theorist determined that statement derivation was indeed needed on the topic of interest. Because the theorist had already identified the two concepts of nurse support and patient coping as the concepts of interest, only a structural linkage was needed for statement derivation. In searching other fields for analogous ways of viewing the nurse-patient interaction during diagnostic procedures, the theorist located literature on the inverted U function. In psychological literature independent variables such as anxiety are related to outcomes such as performance in a curvilinear or inverted U form. Thus, high and low levels of anxiety are related to less effective performance while moderate levels of anxiety are associated with high levels of performance. The inverted U function has proven to be useful in new fields such as interactions between mothers and high-risk infants (Field, 1980). The nurse theorist therefore chose the inverted U function as the "parent" perspective for a statement about nurse support and patient coping. In applying the inverted U function to the concepts of interest, the following statement was derived.

> Nurse support is related to patient coping with pain of intrusive diagnostic procedures as an inverted U function: high and low levels of nurse support are related to low patient coping while moderate levels of nurse support are related to high levels of patient coping.

The inverted U function between nurse support and patient coping is depicted in Figure 8.2.

To complete the statement development process, the theorist then defined key content terms in the derived statement. Nurse support was defined as nurse-uttered sentences not essential to the execution of diagnostic procedures, such as "Relax your forehead," "Count to ten," and "Breathe deeply." Patient coping was defined as absence of distress behaviors such as squirming, teeth gritting, and fist clinching. Although the concepts of nurse support and patient coping were identified by the theorist before beginning statement development, their definitions are included here to give a complete picture of statement development.

In the illustration about nurse support, the theorist utilized only the structural aspect of statement derivation. Because the content concepts were already identified, only a structure for interrelating them was needed. This was provided by the inverted U function.

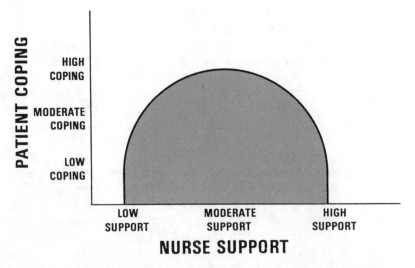

Figure 8.2. Hypothetical Relationship of Nurse Support to Patient Coping During Painful Diagnostic Procedures

Where theorists are deriving both the content and structure of a new statement, the derivation process will resemble the example of family-interaction patterns presented earlier in this chapter.

The derived statement about nurse support predicts how nurse support is related to patient coping. If true, the statement is quite relevant to practice. However, the truthfulness of this or any other derived statements cannot be known before testing. Testing the accuracy of derived statements is quite important to practice. Thus, testing is needed to see if low, moderate, and high levels of nurse support in fact are related to patient coping as an inverted U function. While a lengthy discussion of statement testing is outside the focus of this book, we will indicate links between statement derivation and testing for practice.

Because testing of derived statements is needed before they may be applied with confidence to practice, appropriate methods of testing statements are needed. Several methods that may be used to test derived statements, such as group and single-subject experimental designs and *ex post facto* designs, are presented in Chapter 7. While these methods are described in this book from the viewpoint of statement development, they may be adapted to statement testing with ease. Readers may consult research design references for further information about the use of these designs in a testing context (Baltes et al., 1977; Barlow & Hersen, 1984; Polit & Hungler, 1982; Kerlinger, 1986; Fox, 1982; Campbell & Stanley, 1965; Cook & Campbell, 1979).

An additional way of partially testing derived statements is to examine existing research literature for supporting evidence. Perhaps studies not directly aimed at testing the effects of nurse support in fact contain data that are relevant to the statement in question. Perhaps research has been done in highly related fields such as nurse support with laboring patients. These data, while not a direct test of the support-coping statement, add to its plausibility or nonplausibility. Finally, if highly regarded theories are found to predict the inverted U function between nurse support and coping, a further measure of support is given to the statement. While none of these methods outlined here is a substitute for definitive testing of a derived statement, each aids in making a provisional estimate of the statement's plausibility.

Theorists should not begin evaluating the empirical support for a statement before they have come to closure on the derivation process. Prematurely evaluating the plausibility of a statement may close off the theorist's creative processes. Even in the early stages of derivation when a theorist is selecting parent statements, these should not be stringently judged but simply examined and toyed with. Sometimes seemingly unlikely candidates may prove to be winners in the long run. We are reminded of Maccia and Maccia's (1963) use of the physiology of eye blinking as a framework for deriving statements about student learning. While judging has its place in the context of justification, it should be held in abeyance in the context of discovery (see Chapter 1).

ADVANTAGES AND LIMITATIONS

Statement derivation offers the theorist two advantages. The strategy is an economical and expeditious way of developing statements about a phenomenon. Unlike statement synthesis, the strategy does not require data as a starting point. Armed with only an idea of the phenomenon of interest, reference materials from other fields, and a measure of creative ability, a theorist can accomplish statement derivation. The strategy is not limited to any discipline or phenomenon. It may be used with whatever subject matter a theorist chooses.

Statement derivation has a serious limitation. It is a strategy for discovery, not justification. Thus, derivation of new statements from credible statements in another discipline does not lend support directly to the derived statements. While derivation may facilitate development of interesting new scientific statements, independent empirical support of derived statements is still required. This limitation is, however, not unique to derivation strategies. It applies to synthesis and most analysis strategies as well.

UTILIZING THE RESULTS OF STATEMENT DERIVATION

Because statements generated through the derivation process are essentially untested, their most suitable application is in directing research efforts aimed at testing them. We see two noteworthy areas of research particularly suited for testing derived statements: (1) correlational studies to assess the relationship of an antecedent to a clinical phenomenon and (2) experimental studies to test the usefulness of a nursing intervention to ameliorate a clinical problem. Research methods texts that may be helpful to readers in statement testing are cited earlier in this chapter. To estimate the provisional empirical support for a derived statement, extant research findings often offer clues. For example, correlational data from other studies can sometimes provide information about whether proposed antecedents of clinical phenomena really occur. By examining existing data tables in published research, such provisional evidence can often be located. If found, it supports the need for a research study to directly test the derived statements.

Statement derivation can also be a useful instructional strategy. As a classroom exercise for students, it can be used as the means of generating research hypotheses when students are beginning to learn the research process. Often students get caught up in the details of each specific research topic. Statement derivation offers a means of involving students in joint classroom exercises that free them to think more broadly about phenomena that concern nursing.

SUMMARY

Statement derivation is a strategy that employs an analogy as a basis for constructing new statements about a phenomenon. The theorist selects a parent field as the base for statement development. Analogs in the field to be described are identified. These may occur in the content or structure of derived statements. There are no exact rules for locating fruitful parent fields to use in derivation.

The steps in derivation include becoming familiar with and critiquing literature on the topic of interest, searching for a parent field, identifying content and structural features in parent statements, developing analogous content and structure for derived statements, and redefining new concepts within the new field of interest.

As a strategy, statement derivation is economical and expeditious. Derived statements do require testing independent of the discovery context to establish their empirical validity, that is, "truthfulness."

PRACTICE EXERCISES

Below are statements found in the literature of several disciplines. Before trying to do any derivations with them, identify the phenomenon you would like to derive new statements about. Select one or more of the statements below as a parent statement. Identify the content and structural aspects of the parent statement. Develop the content and structural analogs of the derived statement. Redefine, if needed, any new concepts in the derived statements.

Statements from Several Disciplines

1. The skin provides the most basic and elemental mode of communication—touch (Barnett, 1972, p. 108).

2. The pervasive element of the body's internal environment is the body fluid that bathes the cells of the body and enables the body to leave its ancestral ocean (Snively & Beshear, 1972, p. 3).
3. The more frequently we have made a given response to a given stimulus, the more likely we are to make that response to that stimulus again (Hill, 1963, p. 37).
4. Organisms are surviving because they are adapted, and they are adapted because they are surviving (Burnett & Eisner, 1964, p. v).
5. Neutral events which accompany or precede established negative reinforcements become negatively reinforcing (Skinner, 1953, p. 173).
6. By the preservation of constancy of the internal environment, warm-blooded animals are freed from the influence of vicissitudes in the external environment (Cannon, 1963, p. 178).
7. Blinking functions to protect the eye from contact and to rest the retina and the ocular muscles (Maccia & Maccia, 1963, p. 34).

We will present derivations from two of these statements. Beginning with Statement 7, Maccia and Maccia (1963) derived the following statement about educational processes:

> *Distraction* functions to *protect from mental stress* and to *rest from mental effort* (p. 34).

Words in italics constitute content derivations, while words not italicized represent derived structural forms within which content concepts are located.

In our own derivation exercise, we selected Statement 6. Our wish was to describe the individual's relationship to others with whom social contact is made. We defined the structure of Statement 6 as follows:

> By the preservation of constancy of A, Bs are freed from the influence of C.

We defined the content terms $A-C$ as follows: A is self concept, Bs are human beings, and C is social stressors. By inserting our content terms within the structural form, the following new statement was derived:

> By the preservation of constancy of self concept, human beings are freed from the influence of social stresses.

If you chose to use Statement 6 in your derivations, your content concepts may be quite different from the ones we used.

Compare your derived statements with these examples. While there are no right or wrong derivations, you should be able to identify the content and structural aspects of your derivations and see if they parallel the examples given here. If your derived statements look at all plausible, try to find literature that supports the statements. If you wish, map out a plan for empirically testing your statements.

REFERENCES

Baltes PB, Reese HW, Nesselroade JR: Chapter 23. Developmental research on learning: Single-subject designs. In Life-Span Developmental Psychology: Introduction to Research Methods. Monterey, Calif.: Brooks/Cole, 1977.

Barlow DH, Hersen M: Single-Case Experimental Designs. 2d ed. New York: Pergamon, 1984.

Barnett K: A theoretical construct of the concepts of touch as they relate to nursing. Nurs Res 21: 102–110, 1972.

Burnett AL, Eisner T: Animal Adaptation. New York: Holt, Rinehart & Winston, 1964.

Campbell DT, Stanley JC: Experimental and quasi-experimental designs for research in teaching. In (NL Gage, ed.), Handbook of Research on Teaching. Chicago: Rand McNally, 1965.

Cannon WB: The Wisdom of the Body. New York: Norton, 1963.

Cook TD, Campbell DT: Quasi-Experimentation: Design and Analysis Issues for Field Settings. Boston: Houghton Mifflin, 1979.

Field TM: Interactions of high-risk infants: Quantitative and qualitative differences. In (DB Sawin, RC Hawkins, LO Walker, JH Penticuff, eds.), Exceptional Infant. Vol. 4. Psychosocial Risks in Infant-Environment Transactions. New York: Brunner/Mazel, 1980, 120–143.

Fox D: Fundamentals of Research in Nursing. 4th ed. New York: Appleton-Century-Crofts, 1982.

Hill WF: Learning: A Survey of Psychological Interpretations. San Francisco: Chandler, 1963.

Kerlinger FN: Foundations of Behavioral Research. 3d ed. New York: Holt, Rinehart & Winston, 1986.

Maccia ES, Maccia GS: The way of educational theorizing through models. In (ES Maccia, GS Maccia, & RE Jewett, eds.), Construction of Educational Theory Models. Washington, D. C.: Office of Education, U.S. Department of Health, Education, and Welfare, Cooperative Research Project No. 1632, 1963, 30–45.

Polit DF, Hungler BP: Nursing Research: Principles and Methods. 2d ed. Philadelphia: Lippincott, 1982.

Skinner BF: Science and Human Behavior. New York: Free Press, 1953.

Snively WD, Beshear DR: Textbook of Pathophysiology. Philadelphia: Lippincott, 1972.

ADDITIONAL READINGS

Maccia ES, Maccia GS, Jewett RE (eds.): Construction of Educational Theory Models. Washington, D.C.: Office of Education, U.S. Dept. of Health, Education, and Welfare, Cooperative Research Project No. 1632, 1963.

Maccia ES, Maccia GS: Development of Educational Theory Derived from Three Educational Theory Models. Washington, D. C.: Office of Education, U.S. Dept. of Health, Education, and Welfare, Project No. 5-0638, 1966.

PART IV
Theory Development

INTRODUCTION TO THEORY DEVELOPMENT

Theory development is a very sophisticated and complex level of theorizing, since the theorist must deal with concepts, statements, linkages, and definitions all at the same time. Theory development is greatly needed in nursing, especially the middle-range theory that bridges the gap between the metaparadigm concepts and practice. Using the strategies in the next three chapters should help the theorist to begin appropriate level theory development.

Theory development is needed when one of several situations exists. The first situation in which it is needed is one in which there may be concepts or even relational statements about the theorist's area of interest but no way to link them together. In this case, the most useful strategies might be theory derivation (Chapter 11) or theory synthesis (Chapter 10).

The second situation in which theory development would be needed is one in which there is already theory on the topic of interest. Theory analysis (Chapter 9) would provide the theorist a means of examining the theory to determine its strengths and weaknesses. Once the strengths and weaknesses are known, then further development or testing can be done.

A third situation in which theory development might be needed is one in which there is a body of literature, but it has been unfruitful in suggesting hypotheses for testing or the data it contains are dated or outmoded. In this case any one of the three strategies might be helpful. Theory analysis could indicate deficits and inconsistencies in the current theories. Theory synthesis could provide a means of combining concepts and statements in a new way that could offer insights and provide new hypotheses. And theory derivation could provide concepts and/or a new structure for the concepts that might produce an interesting new unifying idea about the phenomenon of interest.

Asking questions about the level of theory development, the type of literature available on the topic, and the satisfactoriness of the literature will help you decide which strategy will be most useful to you. Theory development is the most challenging pursuit of the scientist, but it is also the most creative and the most fun.

9
Theory Analysis

DEFINITION AND DESCRIPTION

A theory is a set of interrelated relational statements about a phenomenon that is useful for description, explanation, prediction, and control (Hempel, 1965; Reynolds, 1971; Chinn & Jacobs, 1983; Hardy, 1974). It is usually constructed because it expresses a new unifying idea about a phenomenon that answers previously unanswered questions and provides new insights into the nature of the phenomenon. A theory attempts to provide a parsimonious, precise example, or model, of the "real world."

Theory analysis is the systematic examination of the theory for meaning, logical adequacy, usefulness, generality, parsimony, and testability. It is clear that a theory purporting to explain or predict something should provide the reader with a clear idea of what the phenomenon is and does, and what events affect it and how it affects other phenomena.

As in all analysis strategies, the theory is broken into parts. The parts are examined individually and in relation to each other. In addition, the theoretical structure as a whole is examined for such things as validity and approximation to the "real world."

PURPOSES AND USES

There are two basic purposes for theory analysis: to determine the strengths and to determine the weaknesses of the theory. Analysts will usually have one of these two purposes as their primary focus, but both the strengths and the weaknesses of theory need to be examined. In addition, a theory analysis helps determine the need for additional development of the theory.

Theory analysis is useful because it provides a systematic, objective way of examining a theory that may lead to insights and new formulations not seen before. This then adds to the body of knowledge of the discipline. As Popper (1965) has pointed out, science is interested in novel ideas and interesting theories because it is their very novelty or interest that provides the scientist with the impetus to put them to empirical test. Theory analysis is one way of determining "what" needs to be put to the test and often suggests "how" it can be done.

The analyst will probably be interested in conducting a theory analysis only if the theory has the possibility of being useful in either an educational, clinical practice, or research setting. If the theory has no potential for usefulness, then the analyst wastes time in a futile exercise. It has been our experience that the primary purpose for doing a theory analysis prior to using the theory in education and clinical practice has been to discover the strong points the theory offers to guide practice. On the other hand, a theory analysis for the purposes of research usually focuses on the weak points in the theory or the linkages not yet determined between concepts. The reason for this is that the analysis provides the evidence the researcher needs to justify conducting a study on some new or unclear relationships within the theory.

Since a theory analysis is systematic and objective, it provides a way to examine the content and the structure of a theory without becoming involved in valuing the content or structure. Leaving our values out of the analysis allows us to see the theory more clearly, and the original theorist's values will be more evident. The main aim of *analysis* is understanding. To truly understand something one must put aside one's own values and biases and look objectively at the object of analysis. The main aim of *evaluation*, on the other hand, is decision and/or action. At this point, one's own values and biases become important. Evaluation of theory should only be done *after* a thorough analysis is made. At the end of an analysis, the analyst may feel free to and should evaluate the theory's potential contribution to scientific knowledge. Evaluation moves beyond analysis to make judgments about the worth of the theoretical work as a basis for making decisions or taking action (Fawcett, 1980).

PROCEDURES FOR THEORY ANALYSIS

The steps in a theory analysis are (1) to determine the origins of the theory, (2) to examine the meaning of the theory, (3) to analyze the logical adequacy of the theory, (4) to determine the usefulness of the theory, (5) to define the degree of generalizability and the parsimony of the theory, and (6) to determine the testability of the theory. These steps have been synthesized from the works of Popper (1961, 1965), Reynolds (1971), Hardy (1974), Fawcett (1980), and Chinn and Jacobs, (1983). Each of the steps will be defined here briefly and then discussed individually in detail.

The *origins* of a theory refer to the original development of the theory. The analyst will be interested in what prompted its development, whether or not it is inductive or deductive in form, and whether or not there is evidence available to support or refute the theory.

The *meaning* (Hardy, 1974) of a theory has to do with the theory's concepts and how they relate to each other. Essentially, the meaning is reflected in the language of the theory. So examining the meaning implies examining the language the theorist has used.

The *logical adequacy* (Hardy, 1974) of a theory is the logical structure of the concepts and statements independent of the meaning of those concepts or statements. The analyst will be looking for any logical fallacies in the structure of the theory. In addition, the accuracy with which predictions can be made from the theory will be examined.

The *usefulness* of a theory has to do with how practical and helpful the theory is to the discipline in providing a sense of understanding and/or predictable outcomes. A theory that provides a practitioner with realistic guides to practice so that intervention *A* consistently leads to patient behavior *B*, for instance, is more useful than one that does not.

Generalizability refers to the extent to which generalizations can be made from the theory. The more widely the theory can be applied, the more generalizable it is.

Parsimony refers to how simply and briefly a theory can be stated and still be complete in its explanation of the phenomenon in question. Many mathematical theories are parsimonious, for example, because they can express their explanation in only a few equations. Social science theories are rarely parsimonious, on the other hand, because they deal with such complex human phenomena that they defy expression mathematically.

Testability has to do with whether or not the theory can be supported with empirical data. If a theory cannot generate hypotheses that can be subjected to empirical tests through research, it is not testable.

We will now go back and discuss each of these steps more thoroughly and systematically. Remember, each of these steps is important to the theory analysis. We believe that no theory analysis is complete without including all of them. Some authors disagree. Fawcett and Downs (1986) feel that the last four steps—usefulness, generalizability, parsimony, and testability—are really steps in evaluating a theory. However, when you complete the analysis and are ready to evaluate the theory, you may find that you place heavier values on some of the steps than on others. If a theory has poorly defined and inconsistently used concepts, for instance, it will not be capable of test, will not have parsimony, and will not be useful either. The value you assign to a theory will rest primarily on what your analysis reveals, but it will also reflect your own feelings and biases to a certain extent. This is to be expected. No scientist is ever completely objective.

Origins

To analyze a theory, the analyst must first read the theory carefully, identifying the major ideas or concepts and pulling out the relational statements. In addition, the analyst ought to read any research generated by the theory. If the research studies are too numerous, a generous sampling is permissible. Determine from the reading how much research supports and how much refutes the statements in the theory. To do this, look at the hypotheses in the research studies. If they are in the "null" form—that is, stating that there will be no relationship between the variables—and the hypothesis is rejected, it supports the theory (Kerlinger, 1986). If it is accepted, implying no relationship, then it refutes the theory. This sounds confusing, but it is only a function of the way the mathematics work. Rejecting a "null" hypothesis is like stating a double negative in English grammar, two "no's" make a "yes." If the hypotheses are not in the "null" form but actually specify a relationship, then if the hypothesis is rejected it refutes the theory and if it is accepted it supports the theory.

Determine what prompted the development of the theory. Sometimes the theorist will tell you. Otherwise you may only be able to surmise this from the context of the discussion. The origin of a theory and the purpose for which it was developed are often very helpful to the analyst in understanding how the theory was put together and why. In addition, find out if the theory was developed deductively (from a more general law) or inductively (from data). If the theory was developed from another theory or from some other hypothesis, it can be considered deductive in origin. If the theory has been generated by observing relationships from data or from field research or from clinical practice, it can be considered inductive in origin. Later when you are attempting to determine logical adequacy the inductive or deductive form will be important. Once these preliminary activities have taken place you are ready to begin the formal analysis.

Meaning

To analyze the meaning of a theory, one must examine the language of the theory. To do this one must look at the concepts and statements within the theory. The steps are identify the concepts, examine their definitions and use, identify the statements, and examine the relationships between concepts as demonstrated in the statements.

Identify Concepts. To identify the concepts, one looks for the major ideas in the theory. All relevant terms that reflect those ideas should be clearly stated and defined. It is often difficult to identify the major concepts in an elaborate verbal model. Probably the best way to attempt it is to read with a pencil and paper at hand. As new terms appear, write them down with their definitions, if given. This saves time in the long run and makes it very clear where definitions are missing.

When all the concepts have been identified, the next step is to determine what kinds of concepts they are. This involves determining whether they are primitive, concrete, or abstract. As the reader will recall from Chapters 2 and 3, primitive terms are those labels for concepts that derive their meanings from common experience in the discipline and can only be defined by using examples (Wilson, 1969). Concrete concepts are those that are directly measurable and are restricted by time and space. Abstract concepts are those that are not limited by time or space and that may not be directly measurable. Classifying the concepts in this way will give the analyst some clues as to the concreteness or abstractness of the entire theory.

Examine Definitions and Use. Next, one must examine the definitions and uses for the concepts. There are four possible options here in regard to definitions: a theoretical definition, an operational definition, a descriptive definition, and no definition.

A theoretical definition is one that uses other theoretical terms to define the concept. These definitions place the concept within the context of the theory but do not specify any operational rules for classifying or measuring the concept. They are usually fairly abstract and may use lower-order concepts to define higher-order ones. The most important criteria, though, is the lack of measurability of the concept defined.

Operational definitions provide us with the means by which we can classify a phenomenon as an example of the concept or not and also with a means by which to measure the concept in question. Operational definitions are useful for research purposes but often limit the concept artificially. That is, a theoretical definition may provide the theorist with a way of expressing the richness of the concept within the theory, whereas an operational definition would be a severe handicap. It is useful to the analyst, however, if both types of definitions are formulated for the major theoretical concepts. It is also very important to be sure that the operational definitions accurately reflect the theoretical definitions.

The two other definitional options are less helpful to the analyst. A simple descriptive definition, one that simply describes the attributes of a concept, says nothing about the context in which the concept is used, nor does it specify operational measures. It is better than the last option, no definitions at all, but provides very limited data to the analyst. When limited definitions are available, the analyst may find it difficult to get a truly objective analysis and equally difficult to use the theory for the purpose intended. When a theory contains only descriptive definitions or no definitions, it is often in a *very* early stage of development. It will be valuable if the analyst can make thoughtful suggestions about how further development should proceed.

In considering the use to which the concepts are put, the major concern is with consistency of use; that is, whether or not the theorist uses the concepts consistently as they are defined throughout the theory. This is very important to those who propose to use the theory. If a theorist defines a concept in one way and then subtly, or not so subtly, changes the meaning as the theory develops, then all the formulations using that concept become suspect until the ambiguity can be cleared up. Otherwise, one may attempt to predict outcomes from an early statement in a theory only to find that a later statement contradicts those same outcomes.

This is not to say that additional research work with a theory may not cause changes to be made in concept definitions or even in whole sections of a theory. It is to be expected that some refinements should be made. However, when such changes are necessitated, then the initial studies using the original concepts may not be useful in the support of the theory. They may need to be repeated. Neither will the initial relational statements using the concept be considered valid until retested using the new concept definition.

Identify Statements. The third step in analyzing the meaning of a theory is to identify the statements in a theory. The major definitions in the theory should have already been identified and analyzed in the step before this one. Therefore, we will concentrate here specifically on relational statements.

Relational statements are the statements that identify the ways the concepts relate to each other. To identify them is not always easy, especially in elaborate verbal theories. If one is dealing with research reports, one may look in the results section for the major relational statements. At other times, it may be necessary to start with the hypothesis section and work forward to the data analysis in order to find the relationships.

If the analyst is working from a verbal explanation written in non-research-report format, such as a descriptive article or a book chapter, it is often best to look for each concept as it appears and any concepts that lie close to it on the page. Read carefully to see if association between any of the concepts is mentioned. If not, read on until you find some. Often the last few paragraphs or the summary of the article or chapter will offer some relationships, although we have found that summaries often give only the major relationships. Therefore, using summaries alone often leaves much of the richness of the theory in obscurity and hinders the analysis.

Examine Relationships. Examining the relationships between concepts as demonstrated by the statements involves determining what types of relationships are specified, what boundaries are present, and whether the statements are used consistently. In addition, it involves assessing whether or not each statement has any valid empirical support. For the purpose of theory analysis, the question of types of relationships will refer to questions of causation, association, and linearity. (For a more detailed method of statement analysis, the reader is referred to Chapter 6.)

As we have said (see Chapter 6), causal relationships are those that specify that one concept always occurs as a direct result of the other concept. If there is any probability in the relationship whatsoever, it is not a true causal relationship (Hardy, 1974).

Associational relationships are those that specify that two concepts are related positively, negatively, or in no known way. This means that there is correlation between the two concepts but not causation.

A positive association (+) indicates that both concepts vary together; that is, if one is high so is the other. A negative association (−) indicates that as one concept increases, the other concept decreases. When two concepts both occur at the same time but there is no known relationship, the statement is given a question mark (?) to designate it.

In most relational statements, linearity is assumed until proven otherwise. It is by far the easiest relationship to determine and to test. There are other types of relational linkages, however, that can be determined either by deduction or by using data analysis, such as curvilinearity or power curves (Hage, 1972).

Linearity assumes that a change in one variable or concept rather quickly produces an arithmetic change in the other concept or variable. When the correlation coefficient is calculated, the correlation will be strong and the slope of best fit a straight line.

Two other basic forms of relational linkage are found fairly frequently in theories. The most difficult one to determine by analysis is the curvilinear linkage. Curvilinearity assumes that as one concept increases, the other concept also increases until a certain point is reached, and then the second concept begins to decrease. The classic example of curvilinearity is the bell-shaped curve. Another example is the U-shaped curve discussed in Chapter 8. Curvilinearity may be deduced by examining the formal theoretical and relational statements or it may be determined by statistical analysis of data. It is often useful if there are small but significant correlation coefficients among the data, to subject them to nonlinear analysis strategies to determine if perhaps the relationship is nonlinear.

Another kind of relational linkage is the power curve. This type of curve shows an incremental relationship among concepts. That is, if one concept is shown to increase or decrease by a certain amount, the second concept changes at an accelerated rate in either a positive or a negative direction. Power curves are often called exponential curves because the changes in the second concept are often expressed mathematically in terms of exponents. Many of the theories that use "inputs" and "outputs" also use power curves, as do some of the developmental and learning theories. Most power curves represent long time periods (20 years or more) since they must take into account minor fluctuations and individual differences.

The next step in examining relationships involves determining what boundaries are present in the theory. This has to do with the actual content of the theory. Some theories have a very narrow focus and their boundaries, or limits, are very clearly determined. In effect, the theory with narrow boundaries states exactly how far the theory can go in explaining specific phenomena and makes it very clear where the theory starts and stops. For example, a theory would have narrow boundaries if it spoke only to a specific type of preoperative teaching for adults facing abdominal surgery in an American hospital.

A middle-range theory will have wider boundaries and will be more abstract than a narrow theory. The content may be very specific, but the application of it will be to a wider group of events than the narrow theory. An example might be a theory that speaks to several predictable effects from two preoperative teaching strategies on adult surgical patients.

A theory with wide boundaries is highly abstract, covers a large content area, and is applicable in a large number of cases. To extend our preoperative teaching analogy a bit further, a theory with wide boundaries might reflect the effects of any preoperative teaching strategies on any preoperative patients from any cultural background, regardless of age or diagnosis.

To continue examining relationships, determine if the statements are used consistently. This is true of relational statements as well as existence and definitional statements. The theorist should use the statements in exactly the same way at all times. If this is not done, the theory loses credibility and becomes invalid for systematic use.

The last step in examining relationships is to assess the empirical support for the statements. Is there any? If not, the theory will have less validity than one that does. If there is research or empirical evidence to support the statement, the analyst must evaluate the strength of the evidence. A brief series of questions is sufficient to give the analyst a general idea of the validity of the research. These are (Kerlinger, 1986):

1. Do the research hypotheses accurately reflect the theoretical concepts?
2. Is the sampling and sample size adequate?
3. Is the methodology sound and appropriate for the hypothesis proposed?
4. Is the data analysis accurate and appropriate?
5. Are the results reported accurately?
6. Are the conclusions justified?
7. Is the study replicable?

If the answers to these questions are satisfactory, the support is sound. However, if one sound study is good as support for a statement, four or even ten sound studies are that much better. Supporting evidence for a statement must be evaluated quantitatively as well as qualitatively.

Logical Adequacy
Determining the logical adequacy of a theory can get very complicated if one is inclined toward linguistic philosophy, which is based

on formal logic. Since this is basically a strategies book, we will not go as far as the linguistic philosophers. We will limit ourselves to only a few considerations: (1) Is there a system whereby predictions can be made from the theory *independent* of its content? (2) Can scientists in the discipline in which the theory is developed agree on those predictions? (3) Does the actual content make sense? and (4) Are there obvious logical fallacies?

Predictions Independent of Content. In three of our other chapters (Chapters 6, 8, and 10) we have used letters of the alphabet and/or arrows with pluses or minuses over them to denote symbolically how concepts are related to each other. This is precisely the same kind of system that can be used to determine predictions from a theory that are independent of its content. That is, each of the concepts is given a meaningless label such as A, B, or C and then the relationships are diagrammed as are the predictions that can be made from those relationships. This step is important when one is concerned with the logical structure of the theory. If the structure is not logical, predicted relationships may be fallacious. This is not to imply that the content itself is unimportant—only that at this time it is not considered. Content is analyzed in the meaning steps and also in question 3 in this step. If the theory being analyzed cannot be examined in this way, it leaves much to be desired in terms of logical adequacy. This diagramming effort also points out unclear or un-studied relationships among the concepts that are useful for further theory development.

It is often helpful to actually draw a kind of matrix that demonstrates all the specified and unspecified relationships in the theory. Let us examine a theory about the hearing accuracy of a barn owl in this way (Knudsen, 1981). Below are several relational statements from the theory and a matrix to indicate the formal structure.

1. An owl's strike accuracy deteriorates with increases in angle between sound source and head orientation.
2. An owl's ability to locate the origin of a sound is dependent on the presence of high frequencies in the sound.
3. The amount of sound amplification provided by the feathers of the facial ruff varies with the sound frequency.
4. The strike accuracy of the owl increases sharply as the number of frequencies in a sound is increased.

Each of these statements can be written schematically as follows:

1. Strike accuracy (SA) $\xrightarrow{-}$ angle of sound source and head orientation (ASH)

2. Location of origin (*LO*) ± high frequencies in the sound (*HF*)
3. Amount of amplification (*AMP*) ± sound frequencies (*SF*)
4. Strike accuracy (*SA*) ± number of sound frequencies (*SF*)

Once they are written and labels assigned, a matrix may be drawn as we have done in Figure 9.1. The relationships that have been specified in the theory are drawn with solid lines. The relationships that are implied are indicated by dotted lines. All other relationships are unknown.

Another type of matrix that can be drawn is shown in Figure 9.2. This is similar to a correlation table, in which all the variables are listed horizontally as well as vertically and the sign of the relationship is placed in the correct box. Implied relationships are enclosed in parentheses ( ). As you can see, the table is easier to read and the implied relationships can be seen more clearly than in Figure 9.1. Either matrix is acceptable if it helps you get the structure of the relationships clear. If neither is helpful or you feel confused, we refer you to Chapter 6 on statement analysis for additional help or review.

Agreement of Scientists. In addition to being capable of systematic schematic representation, a theory must also be sufficiently precise in its representation for scientists to agree on the predictions that can be made from it. If scientists cannot agree on the possible predictions, the theory is not useful in any scientific sense. If the

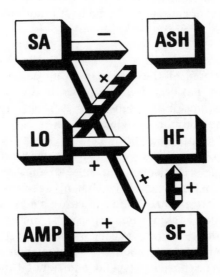

Figure 9.1. Matrix for Statements 1 Through 4 in Text

	SA	LO	AMP	ASH	HF	SF
SA	+	?	?	–	(–)	+
LO		+	?	(+)	+	(+)
AMP			+	?	(+)	+
ASH				+	?	?
HF					+	(+)
SF						+

Figure 9.2. Another Type of Matrix Showing Statements in Figure 9.1

theory is not scientifically useful, it cannot be added to any body of knowledge (except, of course, to the body of knowledge of "things that don't work yet").

Making Sense. Some of the inability to agree on predictions may stem from the fact that occasionally the content of a theory simply is unclear and does not make sense, or it seems to add no useful information to the body of knowledge. This is not to assert that the theory is valueless, although it is certainly less valuable than one that does. It is to assert, however, that a theory may make a great deal of sense to one scientist and no sense to another with a different background. For instance, a theory that makes sense to a maternity nurse may make little sense to one in cardiac care. If scientists with relevant and similar backgrounds all say the theory makes no sense, then it probably doesn't. For a theory to make sense, it must provide insights or understanding about a phenomenon. If it does not, perhaps the theorist needs to spend additional time simplifying or more clearly defining what the theory purports to demonstrate in order to meet the criterion of making sense.

Logical Fallacies. The last step in determining logical adequacy is to look for logical fallacies. This is where the inductive or deductive origins of the theory become important. In a deductive theory, if all the premises are true, then the conclusion, or inference, made from those premises is also true. Therefore, the analyst must determine whether or not the premises of the theory are true. This usually involves a brief review of literature and an evaluation of any supporting evidence to determine the "truth" of the premise. In this case "truth" comes from the validity of the research on which the original premises are based. If the premises are correct then the conclusion will be also.

In an inductive theory, the task is not quite so easy. An inductive inference is usually data-based and can be wrong. In addition, the premises from which the inference is made can be wrong. There are three possible problems with an inductive theory: (1) the premises are correct, but the conclusion is wrong; (2) the premises are incorrect, but the conclusion is correct; or (3) both premises and conclusion are incorrect.

Again, the analyst must return to the literature and to evidence that supports or refutes the premises. In this case the evidence will all be logically inconclusive since the theory is inductive. The analyst will simply have to use the notion of the "preponderance of evidence" to determine the relative truth of the premises. If the evidence strongly supports the premises, one can assume "truth" for the purposes of analysis.

Determining the correctness of the conclusion is more difficult in an inductive theory because the truth of the premises does not guarantee the truth of the conclusion. All the analyst can do here is examine the research that supports the conclusion for validity and determine if the conclusion makes sense given the stated premises and the research evidence. If the conclusion makes sense and if the research is valid and meets all the criteria for a "good" research study, then the analyst is justified in assuming that the conclusion is correct. If the conclusion does not make sense or if the research is poor, no assumptions can be made at all about the conclusion. We simply will not know if the conclusion is correct or not.

Inductive theory is always logically inconclusive, which leaves us always in doubt about the theory's truth. This doubt does not preclude our use of well-supported theory. It only serves to remind us that there may be a better explanation that has not been discovered yet.

The examination of meaning and logical adequacy are the most lengthy processes in a theory analysis. Although the final four steps are not so rigorous or time consuming, they are an important part of a thorough analysis.

Usefulness

Usefulness of theory has to do with how helpful the theory is to the scientist in providing a sense of understanding about the phenomenon in question. If the theory provides new insights into a phenomenon, if it helps the scientist explain the phenomenon better or differently, or if it helps the scientist make better predictions, then it is a useful theory (Berthold, 1968). It adds significantly to the body of knowledge. If the theory does none of these things it is not a useful theory.

To determine the usefulness of a theory, the analyst must consider three issues: (1) How much research has the theory generated (Reynolds, 1971)? (2) To what clinical problem is the theory relevant (Stevens, 1984)? and (3) Does the theory have the potential to influence nursing practice, education, administration, or research (Meleis, 1985)? It is at this point in the analysis that the *content* becomes important. One cannot answer these three questions without considering the content of the theory. If the theory contains subject matter that is already in the scientific domain, it should shed new light on the phenomenon or should provide information that allows clarification, new predictions, or the exertion of control where none previously existed. If the theory covers subject matter that has not been in the scientific domain, it should make some significant difference in that field of science in which it was developed. The theory should generate a significant number of research studies if it is useful. It should be relevant, or at least *potentially* relevant, to a clinical practice setting. It should be capable of influencing, or potentially capable of influencing, nursing practice, education, administration, or research (Meleis, 1985).

Generalizability

The criterion of generalizability refers to how widely the theory can be used in explaining or predicting phenomena. Generalizability can be determined by examining the boundaries of the theory and by evaluating the research that supports the theory. We have said earlier in this chapter that the boundaries of the theory are content related and have to do with how wide the focus of the content is. The wider the focus of a theory, the more generalizable it is likely to be. The more broadly it can be applied, the more generalizable it is.

The research evidence that supports the theory is also important in determining generalizability. If the research evidence is sound, that is, valid and with adequate sample size and reproducible, the theory will be more generalizable than one in which there is little support or the research support is of poor quality. The analyst must have some skills in research critique in order to determine the adequacy of theoretical support. It is not our purpose here to provide those skills, although there are some general questions that can be asked in Chapter 6. In addition, the references at the end of this chapter contain several listings that could be helpful to the reader who perceives a need for additional help.

Parsimony

Parsimony refers to how simple or complex the theory is in explaining the phenomenon it purports to explain. A parsimonious theory is one that is elegant in its simplicity even though it may be broad in its content. Perhaps the best example of parsimony is from Einstein's theory of relativity, $E = mc^2$. This particular statement of the theory revolutionized physics and is very broad in its boundaries but is very simple in its expression. That is parsimony—to explain a complex phenomenon simply and briefly without sacrificing the theory's content, structure, or completeness.

Not all theories are developed to this point. Most theories, especially those in the behavioral sciences, cannot yet be reduced to such a mathematical model. The analyst must examine the theory to see if its formulations are as clear and as brief as they can be. The propositions or relational statements should be precise and should not overlap. If there are several statements, determine if some of them could be reduced to one or two broader, more general, relational statements.

In addition, look for a model or diagram of the theoretical relationships. Many theorists provide models as a way of helping themselves and others visualize the relations of the concepts to each other. If such a model is provided, it should accurately reflect the verbal material in the theory. It must also actually help make the theory clearer. If it does not help clarify the verbal material, it is not a useful model and does not aid in increasing the parsimony of the theory.

Testability

There is some discussion among philosophers of science as to whether or not the criterion of testability is crucial to theory (Hempel, 1965; Popper, 1965; Reynolds, 1971). The debate seems to center on whether or not a theory that provides a great deal of understanding but that by its nature is untestable is a legitimate theory. We do not propose to enter this argument. It seems to us that even a theory that by its nature is untestable as a whole may yield testable hypotheses and relational statements that lend support to the total theory.

We support the idea that for a theory to be truly valid, it must be testable at least in principle. This implies that hypotheses can be generated from the theory, research carried out, and the theory supported by the evidence or modified because of it. A theory that has strong empirical evidence to support it is a stronger theory than one that does not. If a theory cannot generate hypotheses, it is not useful to scientists and does not add to the body of knowledge.

ADVANTAGES AND LIMITATIONS

As in all analysis strategies, the major advantage of theory analysis is the insight into relationships among the concepts and their linkages to each other that the strategy provides. In addition, the analysis strategy allows the theorist to see the strengths of the theory as well as its weaknesses. The theorist is then free to decide whether or not the theory is useful for practice and/or research or whether the theory needs additional testing and validation before use. Where a theory has untested linkages discovered through analysis, it is a spur to the theorist to test those linkages. This both strengthens the theory and adds to the body of knowledge. The major limitation of theory analysis is that analysis only examines parts and their relationship to the whole. It can only expose what is missing, but cannot generate new information. In addition, theory analysis requires evaluation and criticism of supporting evidence. Where the analyst may be limited in the critical skills of research evaluation, important information regarding the soundness of a theory may be disregarded or misinterpreted. This results in a limited analysis and may yield unsatisfactory results.

Theory analysis can provide vital information for the further development of a theory. It is a very helpful strategy for exposing areas that need further work.

UTILIZING THE RESULTS OF THEORY ANALYSIS

We have described the uses of theory analysis as to provide systematic examination of the structure and content of the theory for new insights into a phenomenon and/or to determine its strengths and weaknesses. But what does one do with the analysis when it is completed? The results of theory analysis can be very useful in education, practice, research, and theory development.

In education, the strategy can be used very effectively in the classroom. We have used it successfully to teach students how to examine theories critically. Assigning a theory to a group of students to analyze and then having them report to the class often generates meaningful discussion and debate among the students. Another use of the results of theory analysis is in preparing conceptual frameworks for students' papers. Students have found theory analysis an excellent way to define gaps or inconsistencies in the knowledge about some phenomenon in which they are interested. Yet a third use of the results of theory analysis is in faculty development. As we proposed in the statement analysis chapter, having faculty discussions related to the results of theory analysis on a single topic of interest may generate many useful ideas to be used in curriculum design or in generating faculty research.

In practice, the results of theory analysis may provide the clinician with knowledge about the soundness of any theory being considered for adoption in practice. In addition, knowing which theoretical relationships are well supported provides guidelines for the choice of appropriate interventions and some indications of their efficacy.

Theory analysis is particularly helpful in research because it provides a clear idea of the form and structure of the theory in addition to the relevance of content, and inconsistencies and gaps present. The "missing links," or inconsistencies, are fruitful sources of new research ideas. They also point to the next hypotheses that need to be tested.

The results of theory analysis in theory development are used in much the same ways as in research but with a different focus. In theory development, the inconsistencies, gaps, and "missing links" provide the stimulus to the theorist to keep on working. In addition, the results provide clues to the obvious next steps to be taken to refine the theory.

SUMMARY

Theory analysis is the process of systematically examining a theory for its origins, meaning, logical adequacy, usefulness, generalizability, parsimony, and testability. Each of these seven steps stands alone in a theory analysis and yet each is related to the other. This paradoxical relationship is generated by the act of analysis itself. To do a thorough analysis, one must consider each of the steps, giving them all careful attention. And yet, the results of each of the steps are interdependent on the results of the others.

If concepts are undefined and statements are only definitional in nature, the logical adequacy, usefulness, generalizability, parsimony, and testability of the theory will be affected. If the meaning is adequately handled but the logical structure is missing or fallacious, then usefulness, generalizability, parsimony, and testability will be severely limited. If a theory is not testable and does not generate hypotheses, it is not useful, generalizable, parsimonious, or particularly meaningful. So each step is independent and yet interdependent as well. It is this interdependence that makes the strategy so useful in theory construction. The analysis strategy provides a mechanism for determining the strengths and weaknesses of the theory prior to using it as a guide to practice or in research. With theory analysis, linkages that have not been examined become obvious. This, in turn, should lead to additional testing, thus adding support to the theory or pointing out where modifications need to be made.

Theory analysis is limited in that it does not generate new information outside the confines of the theory. In addition, theory analysis, like all analysis strategies, is rigorous and takes time.

Theory analysis often leads to new insights about the theory being examined, thus adding to the body of knowledge. Finally, theory analysis is one way of promoting additional theory construction by pointing out where additional theoretical work is needed. When pointing out where additional work is needed, it is helpful to remember that comparing anything to the ideal tends to stifle development (Zetterberg, 1965). The best approach is to compare the analyzed theory to similar theories at the same stage of development. To what extent does this theory meet the criteria as compared to others similar to it? Since most theories are generated in the context of discovery, it is more helpful to be encouraging than to be severely critical.

In the next chapter we shall consider theory synthesis, another way of promoting theory construction.

PRACTICE EXERCISE

Reprinted here is an excerpt from Pender's Health Promotion Model. Although Pender does not claim that her model is a theory as yet, it is sufficiently developed to conduct a theory analysis. Pender's model is nearer to a middle-range theory and is therefore very suitable for your practice exercise.

Conduct a theory analysis. When you have completed your own analysis, compare it to the one below. Keep in mind that your analysis will probably be more comprehensive than the one we have included here. Our intention is only to give you clues as to the major strengths and weaknesses of the theory. For those of you who wish to explore this theory further, see Pender's book, *Health Promotion in Nursing Practice*.

When you have completed your analysis, you may compare it with the brief sample that follows Pender's material. Remember that one person's analysis may differ somewhat from another's. They may both be equally valid. The example we have prepared is not a comprehensive analysis. It is only a sample to demonstrate each step.

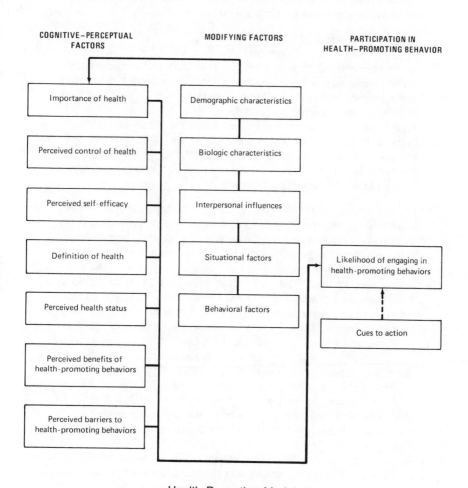

COGNITIVE–PERCEPTUAL FACTORS	MODIFYING FACTORS	PARTICIPATION IN HEALTH–PROMOTING BEHAVIOR

Importance of health

Demographic characteristics

Perceived control of health

Biologic characteristics

Perceived self-efficacy

Interpersonal influences

Definition of health

Situational factors

Likelihood of engaging in health-promoting behaviors

Perceived health status

Behavioral factors

Cues to action

Perceived benefits of health-promoting behaviors

Perceived barriers to health-promoting behaviors

Health Promotion Model

Pender's Health Promotion Model

THE HEALTH PROMOTION MODEL

The Health Promotional Model is derived from social learning theory, which emphasizes the importance of cognitive mediating processes in the regulation of behavior. Structurally, the Health Promotion Model is organized similarly to the Health Belief Model. That is, determinants of health-promoting behavior are categorized into cognitive–perceptual factors (individual perceptions), modifying factors, and variables affecting the likelihood of action. The nature of interrelationships among the variables, additive or multiplicative, will be tested in the research program currently underway.

Cognitive–Perceptual Factors
Cognitive–perceptual factors are identified within the model as the *primary motivational mechanisms* for acquisition and maintenance of health-promoting behaviors. Each factor is proposed as exerting a direct influence on the likelihood of engaging in health-promoting actions. Cognitive–perceptual factors that influence health-promoting behavior have been identified within the model as (1) importance of health, (2) perceived control of health, (3) perceived self-efficacy, (4) definition of health, (5) perceived health status, (6) perceived benefits of health-promoting behavior, and (7) perceived barriers to health-promoting behavior.

The Importance of Health. The impact of valuing health on the frequency of health-promoting behaviors received support from a study of 88 college students conducted by Wallston, Maides, and Wallston. They found that individuals who held a high health value, that is, ranked health within the top 4 out of 10 value positions, chose more health-related pamphlets to read when they were made available to them than did individuals with a low health value. The data support the notion that placing a high value on health results in information-seeking behavior. Thus, individuals engage in actions directed toward becoming more knowledgeable on health-related topics.

Christiansen studied a national probability sample of adults to determine factors that differentiated those engaged in health-promoting activities from those who were not. The importance of health as measured by the Health Value Scale was a significant differentiating factor between persons reporting a moderate to high level of health-promoting behavior and those reporting little health-promoting behavior.

In studying the relationship between value placed on health and participation in physical activity during leisure, Laffrey and Isenberg did not find a significant relationship. The perceived importance of physical exercise per se rather than the value of health was the most powerful variable in explaining exercise behavior.

The role of values in motivating and directing health-promoting behavior needs further study. A person's global value hierarchy may affect the performance of some health behaviors but not others. On the other hand, so many variables may mediate the impact of values on behavior that the relationship is obscured. Behavior-specific values may be more effective predictors of health actions than global life values.

Perceived Control. The effect of perceived personal control on health behavior has been supported in a number of studies. Williams found that individuals who were internally controlled reported more frequent use of seat belts than individuals who were externally controlled. James, Woodruff, and Werner found that nonsmokers were more likely to be internally controlled than smokers, although this finding has been questioned as a result of additional research.

Wallston et al. found that success in weight loss depended on structuring the weight-loss program according to each person's locus of control, either internal or external. Individuals who were externally controlled achieved greater weight loss than internally controlled persons in a group program relying on social pressures as motivation. "Internals" achieved greater weight loss than externally controlled individuals in a self-directed program. Perceived control of health appears to influence the effectiveness of differing strategies for inducing or facilitating continued practice of health-promoting behaviors.

Brown, Muhlenkamp, Fox, and Osborn investigated the relationship between health locus of control, health values, and positive health practices in a sample of 63 middle-class adults in a southwestern metropolitan area. Health locus of control and health values explained 20 percent of the variance in health behaviors. Of the three health locus-of-control dimensions—internality, externality (powerful others), and externality (chance)—only chance explained a significant amount of variance (14 percent) in health practices.

Laffrey and Isenberg, in their study of participation in physical activities during leisure among 75 women between the ages of 24 and 65, found no significant relationship between internal health locus of control and frequency of exercise. Saltzer found that perceptions of health locus of control did not differentiate between persons completing a weight loss program and those who dropped out. However, these groups were distinguished by specific beliefs concerning their ability to control weight. Thus, general health beliefs may be less predictive of health-promoting actions than behavior-specific beliefs.

Desire for control of health and perceived probability of control of health status need to be conceptually and empirically differentiated. Perceiving oneself to be in control as well as having a strong desire for control should result in overt health-promoting behaviors. However, having a strong desire for control but little perceived probability of control may result in helplessness, frustration, and behavioral inhibition. The interactive effects of desire for control and perceptions of control on the occurrence of health-promoting behaviors needs further study.

The importance of cross-cultural investigations on health locus-of-control beliefs is described by Stein, Smith, and Wallston. They pose questions regarding the characteristics of varying cultural environments that may lead to different control desires and expectancies and thus to differential effects of these perceptions on health behaviors.

Perceived Self-Efficacy. Within the revised Health Promotion Model, *desire for competence* has been replaced by *perceived self-efficacy*. While competence represents the generalized ability of an individual to interact or transact effectively with the environment, perceived self-efficacy is a more specific concept that refers to individuals' convictions that they can successfully execute the required behavior necessary to produce a desired outcome.

DiClemente and Condiotte and Lichtenstein found that perceived self-efficacy was an important factor in the maintenance of smoking cessation. They found that perceived inefficacy increased vulnerability to relapse following a period of cessation. At the end of treatment, relapsers as compared to abstainers expressed lower self-efficacy about their ability to resist smoking under subsequent instigating conditions. The higher the perceived self-efficacy, the more successfully smoking cessation was maintained during the follow-up period. Condiotte and Lichtenstein also noted that the highly self-efficacious individuals reinstated control following a slip, whereas the less self-efficacious ones displayed a marked decrease in perceived self-efficacy and relapsed completely. When beset with difficulty, people who have serious doubts about their capabilities often decrease their efforts and give up, while those with a strong sense of efficacy exert greater effort to master problems or challenges.

Chambliss and Murray used persuasion to promote behavior that would increase self-efficacy among persons attempting weight loss. Attribution of efficacy to self had a greater influence on extent of weight loss than perceived locus of control. Atkins, Kaplan, Timms, et al. developed cognitive and behavioral interventions to increase self-efficacy. They used the interventions to determine if the incidence of walking could be increased among persons with chronic obstructive pulmonary disease. Those persons who received the experimental interventions increased in exercise tolerance, reported general health status, and self-efficacy judgments.

Dishman, Sallis, and Orenstein, in reviewing multiple studies on the determinants of physical activity and exercise, concluded that in studies of spontaneous physical activity, there were mixed findings concerning the impact of self-efficacy on exercise frequency. The role of perceptions of self-efficacy in motivating initiation and continuation of health behaviors remains to be demonstrated.

Individuals of all ages are beginning to assume increased responsibility for their own health and to expect greater mastery of personal and environmental factors that impinge on health. It is possible that those people with positive perceptions of their health promotion skills may be more likely to initiate actions that enhance health.

Definition of Health. The definition of health to which individuals subscribe may influence the extent to which they engage in health-promoting behaviors. It is possible that defining health as adaptation

or stability would predispose individuals toward health-protecting behaviors directed toward avoiding illness and disease. Defining health
primarily as self-actualization should result in self-initiated activities
directed toward attaining higher levels of health and well-being.
Since how goals are defined often determines the means used to
achieve them, differences in definitions of health should result in
differing patterns of health behaviors.

The prevailing definition of health within the medical community
is "absence of illness." As the public redefines health as a positive
construct rather than a negative one, the nature of behaviors directed toward maintaining health should also change.

The definition of health to which individuals subscribe was found
by Christiansen to vary greatly from absence of illness to a state of
optimum health and well-being. While Christiansen did not find a
significant relationship between definition of health and frequency of
health-promoting behaviors in the sample she studied, the relationship approached significance. Laffrey developed the Health Conception Scale to measure individuals' definition of health. The scale is
based on the work of Smith, who described four models of health:
clinical, role-performance, adaptive, and eudaimonistic. . . . Laffrey
found that defining health as high-level wellness as opposed to absence of illness was positively correlated with reported participation
in health practices for the purpose of promoting health. Laffrey did
not relate health conception (definition) to the actual frequency of
health behaviors in the sample she studied.

Few studies have focused on the impact of definition of health
on health behaviors. Since personal definitions of health and well-
being appear to be changing in our culture, this area warrants further
study.

Perceived Health Status. Perceived health status appears to play a
role in the frequency and intensity of health-promoting behaviors.
Sidney and Shephard, in studying a group of older adults engaged in
physical training classes for 14 weeks, found that individuals who
exhibited more physical complaints or symptoms on the Cornell
Medical Index Health Questionnaire had a lower frequency and
lower intensity of participation in the exercise program than individuals who reported fewer symptoms on the index. All individuals had
been examined by a physician prior to the program, and any overt
clinical symptoms of illness had been ruled out. The prolonged
experience of uncomfortable symptoms even in the absence of iden-
tifiable illness may represent a threat, induce fear and avoidance,
and reduce personal capacity to engage in positive health behaviors.
"Feeling good" may be a source of motivation for taking actions that
increase personal health status. Kaplan and Cowles have suggested
that an appropriate approach for smoking cessation may be initially
to encourage health-promoting behaviors through which individuals
experience rapid and noticeable changes in well-being, e.g., exercise and relaxation. Experiences of increased well-being and im-

proved health status can then be used to reinforce the value of good health and promote more extensive changes in life style that individuals perceive as difficult.

In a study of 502 individuals between 45 and 69 years of age, Palmore and Luikart found that self-rated health correlated more highly with life satisfaction than did activity level, organizational or social activity, productivity, or career anchorage. Either individuals who are healthy perceive themselves as more satisfied, or self-perceptions of health result in behaviors directed toward achieving increased satisfaction.

Christiansen, in studying a national sample of 378 adults, found that individuals who perceived their health status to be good reported a higher frequency of health-promoting behaviors than individuals who perceived their health status to be poor. Pender and Pender, in studying 377 adults, found that perceived health status was a significant determinant of behavioral intentions to attain or maintain recommended weight. Individuals who perceived themselves to be in good health reported more frequent intentions to control weight than persons reporting that their health status was fair or poor. Dishman et al. concluded from review of studies focused on the determinants of participation in supervised exercise programs that perceptions of being in good health are repeatedly associated with an increased probability of continuing exercise behavior.

Perceived Benefits of Health-Promoting Behaviors. A number of studies have provided evidence that perceived benefits of health-promoting behaviors affect level of participation in such behaviors. In comparing 30 middle-aged males with low-frequency participation in a program of physical activity with 30 males with high-frequency participation, Brunner found marked differences in perceived personal benefits. High-frequency participants ranked keeping fit physically as the most important benefit, while low-frequency participants ranked keeping physically fit fifth in importance. The low-frequency participants ranked the short-term benefit of relaxation at the end of the day as the major benefit of the physical activity program. The data suggest that the perception of long-term benefits rather than short-term benefits from health-promoting behavior may determine frequency of participation and predisposition to continue health-enhancing behaviors.

Sidney and Shephard, in studying 42 elderly men and women participating in supervised physical training, found that individuals who participated more frequently and more intensively than others showed greater awareness of the importance of health and fitness as a benefit and greater appreciation of physical activity as an aesthetic experience. Perception of benefits from health-promoting behavior appears to facilitate continued practice. In addition, repetition of the behavior itself appears to strengthen and reinforce beliefs about benefits.

Perceived Barriers to Health-Promoting Behavior. Within the revised Health Promotion Model, *perceived barriers* has been identified as a cognitive–perceptual factor which, parallel to perceived benefits, exerts a direct influence on predisposition to engage in health-promoting behavior. Barriers to health-promoting behaviors may be imagined or real and consist of perceptions concerning the unavailability, inconvenience, or difficulty of a particular health-promoting option.

A number of studies have supported the importance of barriers as a determinant of frequency of health-promoting behaviors. For instance, inaccessibility of or distance from an exercise facility has been found by a number of investigators to decrease involvement of adults of varying ages in physical fitness activities. Still other investigators found that high intensity of exercise early in physical fitness programs appeared to be a barrier to continuing participation in the program for some individuals who considered the activity too strenuous. Dishman et al. concluded that perceived available time and easy access to facilities were important environmental characteristics that promoted exercise adherence.

Potential or actual barriers to engaging in health-promoting behaviors should be identified for persons of varying ages as well as for families and other aggregates. In addition, the extent to which barriers inhibit specific health behaviors and the adoption of a healthful life style needs further clarification.

Additional Refinements of Cognitive–Perceptual Factors Within the Model. Both self-awareness and self-esteem, components of the Health Promotion Model as originally proposed, have been deleted from the revised model. Self-awareness is a general and rather ambiguous personal characteristic that is not well operationalized. Thus, problems of measuring such a concept are formidable. While the positive impact of self-esteem on physical performance has received some support, there is only limited empirical evidence that self-esteem affects level of participation in health-promoting behaviors. While it may be that individuals who regard themselves highly are more likely to set aside time to nourish personal health than people with low self-esteem, the general rather than specific nature of self-esteem as a personal characteristic may weaken its potential for predicting specific health actions.

Summary. Cognitive–perceptual factors that are proposed in the Health Promotion Model as directly affecting predisposition to engage in health-promoting behaviors include: importance of health, perceived control of health, perceived self-efficacy, definition of health, perceived health status, perceived benefits of health-promoting behaviors, and perceived barriers to health-promoting behaviors. Research is in progress to determine the extent to which the cognitive–perceptual factors identified in the model singly or in additive or multiplicative combination explain exercise habits and life style patterns among adults.

Modifying Factors

Demographic Factors. Characteristics such as age, sex, race, ethnicity, education, and income are proposed within the model as affecting patterns of health-promoting behavior indirectly through their impact on cognitive–perceptual mechanisms. For instance, Sidney and Shephard found that only women identified psychological well-being as an important outcome of exercise, while both men and women believed that improved fitness was a major benefit. Also, when older adults were compared to middle-aged individuals on perceived value of exercise, older adults valued exercise as an aesthetic experience more than the other age group.

In studies of use of preventive services, women rather than men, highly educated versus less well educated, and high-income rather than low-income individuals show more frequent utilization. The extent to which demographic characteristics influence participation in health behavior and the similarities and differences between demographic influences on health-protecting versus health-promoting behavior need to be determined. A closer look at demographic variables and their impact on health actions will clarify critical differences among age, sex, or ethnic groups that must be considered in structuring appropriate health promotion programs.

Biological Characteristics. A number of biological factors have been found to be related to exercise adherence. Pender and Pender found weight to be a significant predictor of intention to engage in exercise. The higher the total body weight, the lower the intention to exercise regularly. In several studies, percent body fat and total body weight discriminated consistently between exercise program adherers and dropouts, with overweight people finding it more difficult to continue with regular exercise when compared to individuals with less body fat or lower weight.

Interpersonal Influences. Interpersonal factors that are proposed within the model as modifying influences on health-promoting behaviors include expectations of significant others, family patterns of health care, and interactions with health professionals. The impact of these factors on health behavior has received support from research findings.

In studying the responses of 239 men to a physical activity program, Heinzelmann found that the expectations of significant others—in this case, the spouses—were important in the men's continuing participation in the program. Although few men reported joining the program primarily as a result of pressure from their wives, positive attitudes toward the program on the part of their wives were critical to continuing participation and program adherence. Eighty percent of those men with wives exhibiting positive attitudes had excellent or good adherence patterns. Only 40 percent of men with wives exhibiting neutral or negative attitudes had excellent or good adherence.

In a study to determine the relative impact of personal attitudes and expectations of others on the occurrence of health-promoting behaviors, Pender and Pender found that exercising regularly was significantly influenced by both factors. Family members, but spouses in particular, exerted an important influence on exercise behavior. Further research is needed to determine the mechanisms through which family members influence participation in health behaviors. The dynamics of family impact on the emergence and continuation of health-enhancing life styles is also an important area for investigation.

Interactions with health professionals constitute another source of interpersonal influence on health-promoting behavior. Sidney and Shephard found that an important reason for participation of the adults that they studied in a physical activity program was the instruction and guidance offered by health professionals. In fact, competent direction of the program by health professionals ranked second in the reasons for participation.

Cox has developed an interactional model of client health behavior that focuses on the interpersonal influence of health professionals on client actions. Empirical testing of the model has indicated its potential usefulness in explaining the occurrence of health behaviors.

Situational Factors. Important situational or environmental determinants of health-promoting behavior appear to include health-promoting options available and ease of access to health-promoting alternatives. The availability of a range of behavioral options increases the opportunity to make responsible choices. For example, if low-cholesterol, low-calorie, or low-sodium meals are not available when one is dining out, there is little opportunity in that situation to behave in a healthful way. Also, if vending machines are stocked with foods high in refined sugars and low in nutritional value, options for healthy behavior by school-age children, industrial workers, and office personnel are limited. Individuals may wish to behave in ways that promote health, but environmental constraints prevent access to healthful options.

Behavioral Factors. Previous experience with health-promoting actions increases the ability of people to carry out various behaviors to promote well-being. Some of the cognitive and psychomotor skills necessary to plan nutritious meals, maintain an exercise program, and deal with stress may have been learned previously from participation in similar activities. Previously acquired knowledge and skills can facilitate the implementation of complex health-promoting behaviors. Dishman et al. identified past physical fitness program participation as a major factor positively influencing current involvement in exercise activities.

Summary. A number of modifying factors are proposed as indirectly influencing patterns of health behavior. These factors include demographic characteristics, biological characteristics, interpersonal influences, situational factors, and behavioral factors. According to the Health Promotion Model, modifying factors exert their influence through the cognitive–perceptual mechanisms that directly affect behavior.

Cues to Action

The likelihood of taking health-promoting action is hypothesized also to depend on activating cues either of internal origin or emanating from the environment. Personal awareness of the potential for growth or increased feelings of well-being from beginning health promotion efforts may serve as important internal cues for behavior. For example, "feeling good" as a result of physical activity can serve as a cue for continuing exercise behavior.

Conversations with others regarding their patterns of exercise, nutrition habits, rest and relaxation, management of stress, and interpersonal relationships can serve as external cues for health promotion. The mass media are a source of cues for action through programs about personal health, family health, and environmental concerns. The intensity of the cues needed to trigger action will depend on the level of readiness of the individual or group to engage in health-promoting activity.

STAGES OF HEALTH BEHAVIOR

A review of health-promotion literature, especially in the areas of exercise and weight loss, suggests there is a distinction between the period of initial involvement in a health-promoting behavior and continuing involvement. A number of health-enhancing behaviors are characterized by a rapid dropout rate within the first 3 to 6 months of initial involvement and a plateau or stabilized dropout rate after that point. This pattern is consistent with a distinction between short-term (1 to 6 months) and long-term (more than 6 months) behavioral stages. Dishman has postulated the existence of distinct adherence stages of health behavior based on several studies suggesting that determinants of health behavior may be different when an expanded time frame is considered. The initial stage of health behavior is referred to by Dishman as the *acquisition stage* and the period of continuation as the *maintenance stage*.

The validity of stage theory is being tested in the research program grant, "Health-Promoting Behavior: Testing a Proposed Model," that was described earlier in this chapter. If differing constellations of cognitive–perceptual factors influence health-promoting behavior during the acquisition and maintenance stages, interventions for facilitating behavior during each stage may differ considerably.

SUMMARY

The Health Promotion Model described in this chapter provides an organizing framework for theory development and research in the area of health-promoting behavior. Literature supporting inclusion of various factors in the revised model is presented. Research that tests the explanatory potential of the Health Promotion Model is in progress. The research program extends over 3 years and consists of projects focusing on working adults, older adults, ambulatory cancer patients, and cardiac rehabilitation clients. Stage theory as proposed by Dishman provides a temporal framework for considering the development and stabilization of health-promoting behaviors. The Health Promotion Model is proposed as an explanation of why individuals engage in health actions. Models to explain health-promoting behaviors of families and communities must yet be developed.

Origins

1. Read theory. Pender states in an earlier portion of the book that the health promotion model was developed as a result of dissatisfaction with several models of health, health beliefs, and primary prevention. She developed her model in an effort to synthesize the features from several of the models that she felt had the most relevance for nursing.
2. Identify major concepts or ideas and relational statements.
   a. Concepts
      (1) cognitive–perceptual factors
         importance of health
         perceived control of health
         perceived self-efficacy
         definition of health
         perceived health status
         perceived benefits of health-promoting behaviors
         perceived barriers to health-promoting behaviors
      (2) modifying factors
         demographic characteristics
         biologic characteristics

        interpersonal influences
        situational factors
        behavioral factors

    (3) likelihood of engaging in health-promoting behaviors

    (4) cues to action

  b. Relational statements

    (1) Cognitive–perceptual factors exert a direct influence on health-promoting behavior.

    (2) Modifying factors indirectly influence patterns of health behavior.

    (3) Health-promoting behavior is influenced by cues to action.

3. Research studies generated by or supporting theory. Each factor in the model is supported by research studies. Pender has been very careful to document the research support for her model.

4. What prompted development? See #1.

5. Purpose of development

  a. To complement models of health protection

6. Formal origin

  a. Based partially on social psychological theory of Lewin as is the Health Belief Model

  b. Primarily inductive. Pender states that the model was developed in part from research findings.

Meaning

1. Identify concepts: see "origins"

2. Examine definitions and use

  a. Some concepts have both theoretical definitions and empirical referents if not operational definitions. Perceived self-efficacy is an example. However, several concepts have only vague definitions that cannot really even be classified as theoretical definitions since they do not contain any defining attributes. The importance of health is one such concept.

  b. Definitions are used consistently.

3. Identify statements: see "origins"

4. Examine relationships

  a. For the three relational statements identified under "origins":

    1 is indicative of a positive relationship.

    2 indicates a positive relationship.

    3 indicates a relationship but no direction is indicated.

  b. The boundaries are relatively wide. The theory is abstract, but it is more like a middle-range theory in that its application is to health promotion only.

  c. The statements are used consistently.

d. There is empirical support for each concept given in the narrative. It is very brief, however, which makes it difficult for the analyst to determine the strength of the evidence.

Logical Adequacy

1. The schematic model gives some indication of relationships that are not specified verbally. For instance, most of the cognitive–perceptual factors as well as the modifying factors appear to be related to each other in the schematic, but these relationships are not dealt with in the narrative. In addition, the modifying factors appear to have a direct effect on the cognitive–perceptual factors, but these relationships are not dealt with in the narrative either.
2. There seems to be sufficient data reported for scientists to agree on many of the proposed relationships. However, it seems to us that several potential relationships are present in the model that have not been addressed by Pender. For instance, it seems that both interpersonal influences and situational factors could have a possible direct effect on health-promotion behaviors, but these relationships are not postulated in the current model.
3. The theory certainly makes sense even with its minor defects.
4. There are not obvious logical fallacies although there are some relationships that are unspecified.

Usefulness
The theory is useful in that it provides a sense of understanding about health-promoting behaviors. It has the potential to provide new insights into the effects of certain variables on the health lifestyles of people. It is limited in that some of its relationships are as yet untested.

Generalizability
The boundaries of this theory are relatively wide but the supporting evidence is accumulating. Even though the theory is abstract it is usable and useful in explaining behavior. The theory has been clinically useful according to Pender and so it is certainly potentially generalizable.

Parsimony
The theory in its current stage of development is more parsimonious than in the first edition of Pender's book. However, it is still in an early stage of development. It may have to get larger before it can become smaller and more elegant.

Testability
The theory is testable but it needs more specific operational definitions for several of the concepts within it. Several studies are currently underway to test the theory according to Pender.

Evaluation
Although this theory is still at a very early stage of development, it seems to be generating a significant amount of research. It still needs operational definitions for several of its concepts, and several of its relationships remain to be clarified. However, it seems to be clinically useful and as such there is hope that this theory will be one of the better first attempts at developing middle-range theory for nursing.

REFERENCES

Berthold FS: Symposium on theory development in nursing. Nurs Res 17(3): 196–197, 1968.

Chinn P, Jacobs M: Theory and Nursing: A Systematic Approach. St. Louis: Mosby, 1983.

Fawcett J: A framework for analysis and evaluation of conceptual models of nursing. Nurs Educ 5(6): 10–14, 1980.

Fawcett J, Downs F: The Relationship of Theory and Research. Norwalk, Conn.: Appleton-Century-Crofts, 1986.

Hage J: Techniques and Problems of Theory Construction in Sociology. New York: John Wiley, 1972.

Hardy M: Theories: Components, development, evaluation. Nurs Res 23(2): 100–106, 1974.

Hempel CG: Aspects of Scientific Explanation. New York: The Free Press, 1965.

Hempel CG: Philosophy of Natural Science. Englewood Cliffs, N.J.: Prentice-Hall, 1966.

Kerlinger F: Foundations of Behavioral Research. 3d ed. New York: Holt, Rinehart & Winston, 1986.

Knudsen EI: The hearing of the barn owl. Sci Amer 245(6): 113–125, 1981.

Meleis A: Theoretical Nursing: Development and Progress. Philadelphia: Lippincott, 1985.

Pender N: Health Promotion in Nursing Practice. 2d ed. Norwalk, Conn: Appleton-Lange, 1987.

Popper KR: Conjectures and Refutations: The Growth of Scientific Knowledge. New York: Harper & Row, 1965.

Popper KR: The Logic of Scientific Discovery. New York: Science Editions, 1961.

Reynolds PD: A Primer in Theory Construction. Indianapolis: Bobbs-Merrill, 1971.

Stevens B: Nursing Theory: Analysis, Application, and Evaluation. Boston: Little, Brown, 1984.

Wilson J: Thinking with Concepts. New York: Cambridge Univ. Press, 1969.

Zetterberg HL: On Theory and Verification in Sociology. Totowa, N.J.: Bedminster Press, 1965.

ADDITIONAL READINGS

Aldous J: Strategies for developing family theory. J Marriage Family 32: 250–257, 1970.

Blalock HM: Theory Construction: From Verbal to Mathematical Formulations. Englewood Cliffs, N.J.: Prentice-Hall, 1969.

Copi I: Introduction to Logic. 7th ed. New York: Macmillan, 1986.

Hanson NR: Patterns of Discovery. London: Cambridge Univ. Press, 1958.

Kaplan A: The Conduct of Inquiry. New York: Chandler Publishing Company, 1964.

10

Theory
Synthesis

INTRODUCTION

Theory synthesis is a strategy aimed at constructing theory, an interrelated system of ideas, from empirical evidence. In this strategy a theorist pulls together available information about a phenomenon. Concepts and statements are organized into a network or whole, a synthesized theory.

Theory synthesis provides a more sophisticated representation of a phenomenon than either concept or statement synthesis. This is true for several reasons. In contrast to concepts, which provide labels for reality, theories demonstrate the connections between concepts. Further, theories simultaneously embrace more aspects of a phenomenon and integrate them more thoroughly than statements. While a statement may link only two or three concepts together (see Figure 10.1a), a theory may connect a number of concepts to each other and also specify complex direct and indirect linkages among concepts (see Figure 10.1b). Theories offer still other benefits. A theory that is well designed moves beyond existing knowledge by pointing the way to new and surprising discoveries (Causey, 1969; Hempel, 1966, pp. 70–84).

Synthesized theories may be expressed in several ways. When the relationships within and among statements are depicted in graphic form, this constitutes a *model* of the phenomenon (see Chapter 2 on the terminology of theory construction). In this chapter we will use the terms *theory* and *theoretical model* interchangeably because it is often quite useful to represent beginning theories in both

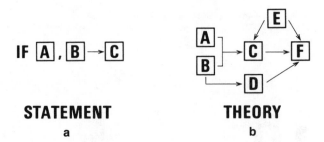

STATEMENT   **THEORY**

a   b

Figure 10.1. Example of Complexity of Linkages in Statement (**a**) Versus Theory (**b**)

graphic (model) and linguistic (theory) form. Theorists often move back and forth between expressing theories in written sentences and visual devices, such as diagrams, during theory construction. In the final stages of theory building and refinement, theories may also be expressed in mathematical form (Blalock, 1969). Here, given that this is an introductory book on theory construction, we will limit ourselves to linguistic and graphic expressions of theory.

Theory synthesis, like other synthesis strategies, builds on a base of empirical evidence. In theory synthesis, a theorist may combine information from various sources during theory building: field observations, available data banks, and published research findings. In utilizing field observations and statistical information in theory synthesis, it is helpful to first translate them into statement form (see Chapter 7). Because a theorist can use a variety of sources of data in theory synthesis, we will not present distinct methods for each source. Rather, we will attend to each source of data within an overall strategy for theory synthesis. A theorist might then utilize evidence from each of these sources in the construction of a particular model. In theory synthesis the source of data is less important than the salience of the evidence to the phenomenon represented by the model.

Like other synthesis strategies, a synthesized theory is limited in its generalizability or external validity by the extent and quality of evidence upon which it is based. Theoretical models drawn from a limited number of sources will generally be more restricted in focus and less generalizable than ones based on multiple and diverse sources. Synthesis strategies are more "grounded" in reality, however, than other strategies such as derivation, because they are in fact based on real data. Synthesized theories, like synthesized statements, require testing or cross-validating to reaffirm their empirical validity.

An understanding of statistical concepts is a valuable tool in theory synthesis. Knowledge of statistics enables a theorist to directly utilize statistical information to which they have access in theory construction. Further, theorists who are conversant in statistics are better able to critically evaluate the accuracy of statements based on others' statistical findings. While knowledge of statistics is not absolutely essential for doing theory synthesis, theorists without such knowledge are well advised to seek consultation about statistical matters they encounter in theory synthesis.

We will limit our use of statistical information to an introductory level in this chapter. Readers who wish to quickly assess their knowledge of introductory statistics may complete the pretest at the end of Chapter 7. References on introductory statistics are also at the end of Chapter 7. For interested readers we have provided a brief listing of advanced statistical references at the end of this chapter. Readers with an advanced knowledge of statistics will no doubt see the greater precision that statistical procedures such as part and partial correlation, multiple regression, and factor analysis can contribute to model construction.

Because it is probably easiest to get a grasp on how theory synthesis works by demonstrating the process, we provide the illustration that follows. Highlights of a review of research findings on stress in critical care nursing are given (Stehle, 1981). We focused selectively on findings drawn from the intensive care unit (ICU). Readers who find the topic of particular interest are referred to Stehle's original article for more complete details of how the review was done and its conclusions. [Note, we have identified each finding about factors related to nurse stress by assigning an alphabetical letter (A, B, etc.) to it. These letters are also included in the model we constructed from Stehle's literature review, Figure 10.2, so that readers may trace the translation we made from linguistic to graphic representation of the findings.]

Studies of stress in critical care nursing settings reported that staff rotation (A), intense emotions in interpersonal situations (B), complicated machinery (C), narrow patient focus (D), great responsibility (E), conflict with administration (F), and crisis atmosphere (G) were related to nurse stress in the ICU. ICU nurses' major defense mechanism for adapting to stress is denial of stress (H). Somatic symptoms, such as tachycardia, in ICU nurses was also suggested as responses to stress (I). Despite limited and unclear findings about the relationship between nurses' personalities and stress in the ICU (J), it appears at this point that stress is more dependent on environmental factors (A–G) than intrapersonal ones (J). While Stehle reported conflicting findings, there is some evidence that stress in the ICU is

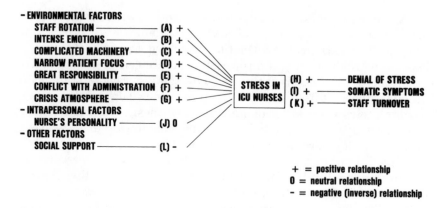

Figure 10.2. Factors Related to Stress in ICU Nurses. *Based on selected information extracted from Stehle (1981).*

related to staff turnover (*K*). Having identified a series of relationships pertinent to stress among ICU nurses, we then constructed a diagram, Figure 10.2, to represent the relationships as an interrelated network of ideas. To Stehle's listing of factors, we added a further one that we believed to be important although it is not directly based on studying ICU nurses: social support may moderate the effects of stress (*L*). Although there are criticisms of *L*, for example, Heller (1979), the statement is supported by a wide body of research literature (Cobb, 1976) and thus seemed very pertinent to us.

In constructing Figure 10.2, the symbols +, 0, and − were used to designate respectively factors with positive, neutral, and negative relationships to stress in ICU nurses. While Stehle's review did not directly address the issues of causality and direction of influence among factors associated vith stress in ICU nurses, we treated the relationships as unidirectional and causal in our illustration by using the symbol → (see Chapter 7 for further discussion of the concepts of directionality and causality).

Further research and review are needed to determine if our assumptions about causality and directionality were correct. One important limitation of Stehle's review and our accompanying model is that interrelationships among stressors are not addressed: Are staff rotation and intensive emotions related to each other in addition to their individual relationships of nurse stress? Further, possible relationships among the effects or outcomes of stress are also not considered. Are the effects of stress such as somatic symptoms and turnover related? Careful review of literature and further research are needed to answer these kinds of questions about the proposed model of stress in nurses.

In our example of ICU nursing stress, our synthesized model or theory was based on reported research findings. We could have also drawn factors from other sources. For example, while the illustration did not involve direct statistical information, this is not always the case. Had we had access to a data bank on ICU nurses we might have generated further information pertinent to the model constructed. Suppose we had done this and found that stress was correlated ($r = 0.50$) with changes in life-style of nurses in the preceding six months. We would then have added changes in life-style as a factor leading to ICU nursing stress. Statistical information translated into a statement of relationship may be entered into a theoretical model in the same way as relationships gleaned from the literature.

PURPOSE AND USES

The general purpose of theory synthesis is to represent a phenomenon through an interrelated set of concepts and statements. Several more specific purposes for theory synthesis include (1) to represent the factors that precede or influence a particular event, such as factors that lead to resuming work roles after a heart attack; (2) to represent effects that occur after some event, such as changes in health behaviors after receiving patient education; or (3) to simply put discrete scientific information into a more theoretically organized form. Using theory synthesis for this third purpose involves organizing relational statements into a system and collapsing factors or variables that resemble each other into larger summary concepts. Conducting theory synthesis for this last purpose is less concerned with depicting relationships about a phenomenon than focusing on improving the overall form and quality with which a theory is expressed. In contrast, the first purpose may be especially directed to predicting and perhaps controlling some clinical event. The second is similarly helpful in predicting and controlling effects that are desired or undesired consequences of a clinical phenomenon. The varied purposes of theory synthesis are equally valid. The specific purpose for which a theorist engages in theory synthesis will depend on the interests of the theorist and the use envisioned for the synthesized theory.

Still a further consideration in delineating the purpose of theory synthesis is the nature of available evidence. If only minimal information is available about the effects of some event but a great deal is known about antecedents or determinants of the event, a theorist simply has more information to work with if antecedents are chosen as the focus for theory synthesis. There must generally be research evidence available about relationships among at least three factors, at a minimum, for theory synthesis to be possible. If this is not the case, the theorist should consider another strategy, for example, statement synthesis or theory derivation. The richer the pool of research information available to the theorist, the greater the complexity and precision possible in a synthesized theory.

Theory synthesis is applicable in a wide range of both scientific and practical situations. Theory synthesis can be used to produce a compact high-information-content graphic representation of research findings on a topic of interest (see Figure 10.2). Literature reviews about multiple and complex relationships may be made less tedious and more informative through theory synthesis. Particularly where a graphic display of a synthesized theory is made, complex relations may be communicated more effectively than through traditional written reviews. This particular use of theory synthesis is relevant in the teaching of complex content about a clinical topic, applying research to the design of clinical interventions, and developing a theoretical framework for a research project.

Because theory synthesis requires that a theorist systematically assess relationships between factors pertinent to a topic of interest, the process aids in highlighting areas in need of further research. As the theorist methodically identifies relationships between variables; notes the directionality of the relationships; specifies whether the relationship is positive, neutral, or negative; and notes the quality and amount of evidence in support of the relationship; over-researched and under-researched areas become patent. This information can be helpful in locating specific questions in need of investigation. [See Schwirian (1981) for an example of theory synthesis used in this way.]

PROCEDURES FOR THEORY SYNTHESIS

Although theory synthesis may be used for several purposes, a common set of procedures comprises theory synthesis regardless of purpose. While we will outline the procedures as a set of steps, their order is not absolute nor will a theorist necessarily devote comparable time to each.

1. To begin theory synthesis, a theorist must mark off a topic of interest. The theorist may do this by specifying (a) *one focal concept* or variable, such as Stehle's concept of ICU nursing stress, or (b) a *framework* of several focal concepts. In the former case, the theorist

moves out from the focal concept, for example, nurse stress, to other concepts or variables related to it. In the latter case, the theorist is concerned with a framework of focal concepts and how they may be interrelated. For example, the relationship of various teacher attitudes and behaviors to various student attitudes and behaviors constitutes a framework of focal concepts for beginning theory synthesis.

2. Using either a single focal concept or a framework of concepts as an entry point into the literature, a careful review is done next. During the review, note is taken of variables related to the focal concept or framework of concepts. Relationships identified are systematically recorded indicating, where possible, whether they are bi- or unidirectional; positive, neutral, or negative; and weak, ambiguous, or strong in supporting evidence. Locating relationships in research may be facilitated by finding comprehensive and thorough review articles already written. If recent reviews on the focal concepts are not available, a thorough search of the literature is in order. Relationship statements are not located in one uniform place in research articles and reports. They may be clearly stated in the summary of results or discussion section. If the results of a study are not presented in clear statements, a theorist may have to trace a statement from the hypothesis section through the results section in order to determine if it was supported by actual findings of the study.

Step 2 may also be expanded to include other than literary sources of statements and concepts, for example, direct statistical information and field observations made by the theorist. As indicated earlier in this chapter, direct statistical information is translated into relational statements and then treated as any other statement in theory synthesis. If theorists wish to utilize observations made in the field, these may be constructed from the theorist's memory and field notes into statements of relationships. Statements and concepts drawn from field observations are also incorporated into theoretical models in the same manner as any other empirically based statement.

3. When a theorist has collected a fairly representative listing of relational statements pertinent to one or more focal concepts, these may then be organized in terms of the overall pattern of relationships among variables. Diagrams are particularly helpful in expressing relationships among concepts and constitute the major device a theorist may use at this step to organize material. Readers will recall that the ICU nursing stress illustration organized variables into those that appeared to lead to stress and those that appeared to be effects of stress (see Figure 10.2). For each topic of interest a theorist must determine what is a reasonable basis for organizing statements.

Zetterberg (1965) introduced the terms "inventory of determinants" and "inventory of results" to refer respectively to the cataloging of antecedents and effects of a focal concept or variable. Structurally, these two types of inventories are quite similar. They differ only in whether the focal concept is viewed as an outcome of certain variables or a determinant of them (see Figure 10.3). Organizing statements into inventories of determinants and results is often helpful where a theorist is dealing with only one focal concept or variable.

Blalock (1969) recommended organizing sets of variables into theoretical "blocks." With this approach, variables that are more proximally related are organized together into a "block" and their interrelationships specified. Each block of variables is then related to more distally related variables in other blocks (see Figure 10.4). Organizing variables and relationships into theoretical blocks is especially relevant if a theorist is constructing a "megamodel" comprised of several "minimodels." In Figure 10.5, we present an application of Blalock's blocking method applied to nursing. Schwirian (1981) pulled together a large body of research findings on nursing performance. Individual variables were then sorted into seven theoretical blocks: academic achievement, demographic characteristics, personal characteristics, employment characteristics, family of origin characteristics, nursing school characteristics, and nurse career behavior. Relationships were specified both within and between blocks of variables.

One final method that may be used to organize variables is to collapse several highly similar variables into a more comprehensive

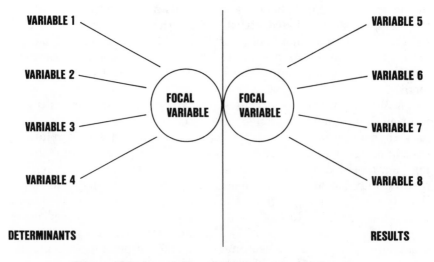

Figure 10.3. Inventories of Determinants and Results

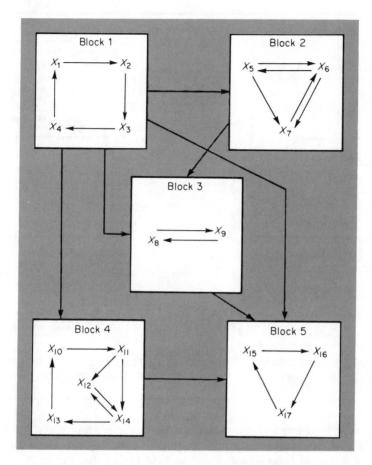

Figure 10.4. Variables and Statements Organized into Theoretical Blocks. *From Hubert M. Blalock, Theory Construction: From Verbal to Mathematical Formulations, © 1968, p. 72. Reprinted by permission of Prentice-Hall, Inc., Englewood Cliffs, N. J.*

summary concept. For example, smiling, kissing, and cuddling might all be amalgamated into a summary concept of affectionate behavior. Similarly, return to work, normal blood sugar, and absence of sugar in urine may be collapsed under the concept of adaptation to chronic disease. Collapsing discrete variables into summary variables can make a theory more easily understood by reducing needless complexity. A more parsimonious theory will also be achieved by this method. Readers may find Chapter 4 on concept synthesis helpful in constructing summary concepts.

These three steps comprise the basic maneuvers of theory synthesis. As mentioned earlier, the order of these steps is not absolute.

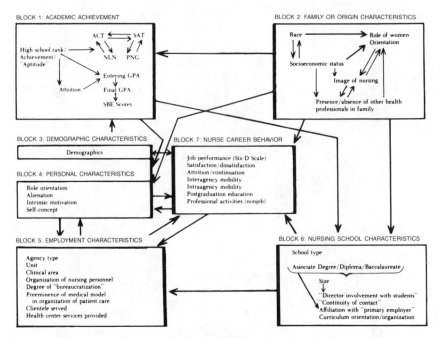

Figure 10.5. Model of Nurse Performance Organized by Blocks. *From Schwirian, PM: Toward an explanatory model of nursing performance, Nurs Res 30: 248, 1981.*

They may be varied or expanded as needed. For example, conducting the literature review (step 2) may be necessary to help theorists clarify the focal concepts of greatest interest to them (step 1). Step 3 may be embellished by diagrammatically organizing concepts and relational statements and then further coding them as to the extent of research support (*** = high support, * = low support, ? = conflicting support).

To illustrate the steps of theory synthesis, we will present the model of adherence among hypertensive patients constructed by Caplan et al. (1976). Caplan and others began model construction by specifying the major dependent variables of interest: adherence and the lowering of blood pressure. They then proceeded to work backwards to identify predictors or determinants of these focal variables. In constructing the model they expressed the hope that it would "serve as a heuristic aid in thinking about determinants of adherence" (p. 22). Below are key statements, largely paraphrased for brevity, that culminated in the Caplan et al. model.

Medical evidence supports the relationships between maintaining blood pressure in normal limits and the goal of longevity, if not a long satisfying life (A). Adherence to medical regimens that involve, most importantly, taking medications is an effective means of controlling high blood pressure (B). In attaining adherence, setting specific subgoals is important in goal attainment, and "rewards need to be anticipated, or explicitly identified in advance before the person begins to strive toward the goal" (p. 26) to meet the desired level of adherence (D). Further, patients' actual adherent behaviors "serve as a feedback mechanism helping them set new goals based on past accomplishments" (D) (p. 30). Accomplishment enhances patients' perceived competence to adhere (E). Perceived competence to adhere leads to further adherence behavior (C).

Caplan et al. represented these relational statements in graphic form (see Figure 10.6). As with the nurse stress illustration, letters are used to connect relational statements in linguistic form with their translation into graphic form. Of note in the Caplan et al. model is the bidirectional relationship between adherent behavior and goal setting and attainment (D). Two subsequent expansions of this model were made by Caplan et al. (1976), but for brevity we have not included those here.

The theoretical models of nursing stress, nursing performance, and finally, adherence among hypertensive patients demonstrate that synthesized theories may take a variety of forms. These forms may often be guided by structural "blueprints" such as Zetterberg's inventories of determinants and results and Blalock's theoretical blocks. While such blueprints can be quite useful, theorists should

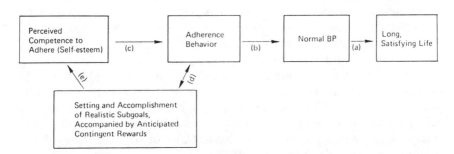

Figure 10.6. Model of Major Hypothesized Predictors of Adherence and Their Effects on Blood Pressure. Arrows between boxes indicate causal relationships. The letters on each arrow are used for reference in the text. *From Caplan RD, Robinson EAR, French JRP, Caldwell JR, Shinn M: Adhering to Medical Regimens: Pilot Experiments in Patient Education and Social Support. Ann Arbor, Mich.: Institute for Social Research, Univ. of Michigan, 1976, 21.*

not be blinded by their elegance. Superimposing an elegant blueprint upon a body of literature for which it is ill-fitted is counterproductive. In the end, theorists themselves must decide on the most accurate and meaningful ways to organize statements and concepts into theoretical models.

Before leaving procedures for theory synthesis, we must note that even a well-designed theoretical model needs to be empirically validated. Model or theory testing are needed to provide the sound empirical base desired of theories in a scientific discipline and profession. Testing of large-scale theoretical models is only beginning in nursing (e.g., Munro, 1980). While there are prototypes for model testing in other disciplines (e.g., Kerlinger and Pedhazur, 1973, pp. 433–441), further design and execution of model testing programs are essential for the continued growth and improvement of theory in nursing.

ADVANTAGES AND LIMITATIONS

Theory synthesis is a valuable strategy for integrating large amounts of discrete information about a topic. By using both linguistic and graphic modalities, synthesized theories can integrate and efficiently present multiple and complex relationships. Theory synthesis is a useful strategy for summarizing research findings relevant to educational, research, and practice spheres.

Where theorists are limited in their fluency with statistical concepts, important discriminations about structural relationships between and among concepts in a theory (Field, 1979) are precluded. These discriminations include clarifying causal pathways among sets of variables. Some of these discriminations can be made, however, if theorists seek and maintain competent statistical consultants in their theory-building programs.

Theory synthesis implicitly proceeds on the premise that theory development is an incremental and cumulative process. While this may be true at certain levels of scientific development, this may not characterize those major advances in scientific thought that have occurred by making radical reorganizations of or departures from accumulated knowledge (Kuhn, 1962).

UTILIZING THE RESULTS OF THEORY SYNTHESIS

The results of theory synthesis have applicability to research, education, and practice. For research, theory synthesis results lay bare the conceptual structure and linkages of extant knowledge about a phenomenon. This structural knowledge may then be used to ensure operational adequacy (Fawcett & Downs, 1986) of indicators and research procedures in empirically testing synthesized theory.

In education, synthesized theories may be useful in teaching complex content involving multiple concepts and their interrelationships. Often when such material is presented graphically and linguistically, it is easier both to teach and learn.

While it is unlikely that many nurses in practice would find synthesized theories immediately useful in their day-to-day work, such theories may offer some utility if new programs or reevaluations of ongoing programs are needed. Examining the antecedents and consequences of a clinical phenomenon may help to show areas that have been neglected in planning programs or services. Designing preventive interventions may also be facilitated by looking at the antecedents of a clinical problem. Tracing the way that each potential antecedent might be modified in an attempt to prevent undesired clinical problems, such as hospital readmissions after surgery, can suggest how present practice might be improved. This approach is also applicable to clinical problems outside the hospital context, as in home care and community agency settings.

SUMMARY

Theory synthesis, a strategy based on empirical evidence, enables a theorist to organize and integrate a wide variety of research information on a topic of interest. In theory synthesis sets of concepts and discrete statements are organized into an interrelated system of statements with accompaning graphic representations. Theory synthesis may incorporate information from published research literature, direct statistical information, and field observations. Because theory synthesis may be used for several related purposes, deciding on the specific purpose depends on the balance among the theorist's interests, the use planned for the synthesized theory, and the amount and type of information available on a topic.

Theory synthesis includes three basic steps: (1) specifying focal concepts for the synthesized theory, (2) reviewing the literature to identify factors related to the focal variables or concepts and the relationships between these, and (3) organizing concepts and statements about a phenomenon into an integrated and efficient representation of it.

With theory synthesis a large amount of information can be efficiently organized. The use of the method may be limited somewhat by the statistical sophistication of the theorist and the inherent assumptions of the method about the nature of scientific progress.

PRACTICE EXERCISE

For the practice exercise, we have drawn together a listing of statements relevant to the focal concept of infant attachment. The statements are listed below. After reading the statements, decide on a plan to organize them. Arrange the statements according to plan and prepare a diagram consistent with the plan.

Statements about Infant Attachment

1. Attachment is positively related to the amount of love and caretaking provided by the mother and the immediacy of her response to supplication (Sears, 1972).
2. Attachment is evidenced immediately by proximity-seeking, visual contact, and pleasure and contact following brief separation (Ainsworth et al., 1978).
3. Attachment in infancy is related to later problem-solving behavior, curiosity, and ego resiliency (Matas et al., 1978; Arend et al., 1979).

When you have completed this exercise, compare your theoretical model with Figure 10.7. This figure presents a model that we consider a reasonable representation of statements 1–3. While your model may not look exactly like ours, there should be some structural similarity to it.

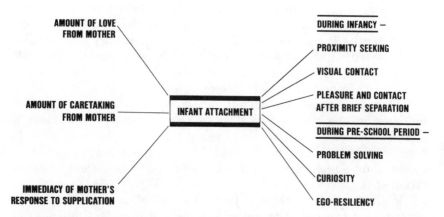

Figure 10.7. Model of Determinants and Effects of Infant Attachment

REFERENCES

Ainsworth MDS, Blehar MC, Waters E, Wall S: Patterns of Attachment: A Psychological Study of the Strange Situation. Hillsdale, N.J.: Erlbaum, 1978.

Arend R, Gove FL, Stroufe LA: Continuity of individual adaptation from infancy to kindergarten: A predictive study of ego-resiliency and curiosity in preschoolers. Child Dev 50: 950–959, 1979.

Blalock HM: Theory Construction: From Verbal to Mathematical Formulations. Englewood Cliffs, N.J.: Prentice-Hall, 1969.

Caplan RD, Robinson EAR, French JRP, Caldwell JR, Shinn M: Adhering to Medical Regimens: Pilot experiments in Patient Education and Social Support. Ann Arbor, Mich.: Inst. for Social Research, Univ. of Michigan, 1976.

Causey R: Scientific progress. Tex Eng Sci Mag 6(1): 22–29, 1969.

Cobb S: Social support as a moderator of life stress. Psychosom Med 38: 300–314, 1976.

Fawcett J, Downs FS: The Relationship of Theory and Research. Norwalk, Conn.: Appleton-Century-Crofts, 1986.

Field M: Causal inferences in behavioral research. Adv Nurs Sci 2(1): 81–93, 1979.

Heller K: The effects of social support: Prevention and treatment implications. In (AP Goldstein & FH Kanfer, eds.), Maximizing Treatment Gains. New York: Academic Press, 1979.

Hempel CG: Philosophy of Natural Science. Englewood Cliffs, N.J.: Prentice-Hall, 1966.

Kerlinger FN, Pedhazur EJ: Multiple Regression in Behavioral Research. New York: Holt, Rinehart & Winston, 1973.

Kuhn TS: The Structure of Scientific Revolutions. Chicago: Univ. of Chicago Press, 1962.

Matas L, Arend RA, Sroufe LA: Continuity of adaptation in the second year: The relationship between quality of attachment and later competence. Child Dev 49: 547–556, 1978.

Munro BH: Dropouts from nursing education: Path analysis of a national sample. Nurs Res 29: 371–377, 1980.

Schwirian PM: Toward an explanatory model of nursing performance. Nurs Res 30: 247–253, 1981.

Sears RR: Attachment, dependency, and frustration. In (JL Gewirtz, ed.), Attachment and dependency. New York: John Wiley, 1972.

Stehle JL: Critical care nursing stress: The findings revisited. Nurs Res 30: 182–186, 1981.

Zetterberg HL: On Theory and Verification in Sociology. Totowa, N.J.: Bedminster Press, 1965.

ADDITIONAL READINGS

Readings in Advanced Statistics

References preceded by an * utilize primarily a conceptual approach to statistics.

*Achenbach TM: Chapter 6. Multivariate statistics. In Research in Developmental Psychology: Concepts, Strategies, Methods. New York: Free Press, 1978.

Duncan OD: Introduction to Structural Equation Models. New York: Academic Press, 1975.
Glass GV, Hopkins KD: Statistical Methods in Education and Psychology. 2d ed. Englewood Cliffs, N.J.: Prentice-Hall, 1984.
Hays WL: Statistics. 3d ed. New York: Holt, Rinehart & Winston, 1981.
Hollander M, Wolfe DA: Nonparametric Statistical Methods. New York: John Wiley, 1973.
Kerlinger FN: Foundations of Behavioral Research. 3d ed. New York: Holt, Rinehart & Winston, 1986.
Kerlinger FN, Pedhazur EJ: Multiple Regression in Behavioral Research. New York: Holt, Rinehart & Winston, 1973.
Tabachnick BG, Fidell LS: Using Multivariate Statistics. Philadelphia: Harper & Row, 1983.

Readings in Theory Development

Blalock HM: Theory Construction: From Verbal to Mathematical Formulations. Englewood Cliffs, N.J.: Prentice-Hall, 1969.
Dubin R: Theory Building. New York: Free Press, 1978.
Hage J: Techniques and Problems of Theory Construction in Sociology. New York: John Wiley, 1972.
Lancaster W, Lancaster J: Models and model building in nursing. Adv Nurs Sci 3(3): 31–42, 1981.
Mullins NC: The Art of Theory: Construction and Use. New York: Harper & Row, 1971.
Reynolds PD: A Primer in Theory Construction. Indianapolis: Bobbs-Merrill, 1971.
Stember ML: Model building as a strategy for theory development. In (PL Chinn, ed.), Nursing Research Methodology. Rockville, Md.: Aspen, 1986.
Zetterberg HL: On Theory and Verification in Sociology. Totowa, N.J.: Bedminster Press, 1965.

11

Theory
Derivation

DEFINITION AND DESCRIPTION

Theory derivation is the process of using analogy to obtain explanations or predictions about a phenomenon in one field from the explanations or predictions in another field (Maccia and Maccia, 1963).
Thus, a theory (T_1) from one field of interest (F_1) offers some new
insights to a theorist who then moves certain content or structural
features into his or her own field of interest (F_2) to form a new theory
(T_2). Theory derivation is an easy way to develop theory rapidly in a
new field since all that is required is (1) the ability to see analogous
dimensions of phenomena in two distinct fields of interest and (2) the
ability to redefine and transpose the content and/or structure from
Field 1 to Field 2 in a manner that adds significant insights about
some phenomenon in Field 2 (see Figure 11.1).

Theory derivation is not a mechanical exercise. Seeing the analogy requires imagination and creativity. Theory derivation also requires the theorist to be able to redefine the concepts and statements

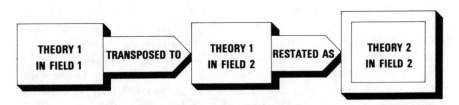

Figure 11.1. Process of Theory Derivation

so that they are meaningful in the new field. Since the two fields are obviously different, certain modifications will have to be made when transposing a theory from one to the other field.

Two distinctions must be made here: the distinction between theory derivation and statement derivation, and the distinction between "borrowing" theory and theory derivation. Theory derivation is a process whereby a whole set of interrelated concepts or a whole structure is moved from one field to another and modified to fit the new field, whereas in statement derivation one moves only *individual* isolated statements from one field to another and modifies them. Statement derivation is on a smaller scale than theory derivation although the actual steps in the process are similar.

Borrowing theory is a practice that nurses have used frequently. When one borrows a theory, the theory is moved *unchanged* from one discipline to another. For example, we have used chemical, biological, and psychological theories in nursing for many years without any changes needing to be made in the original theories when they are applied in nursing. However, if we wished to *derive* a new theory to use in nursing from any of these fields, we would need to modify the concepts and/or the structure in those theories to fit our particular needs in nursing. Theories cannot be moved unchanged from one field to another as an example of theory derivation. True theory derivation requires that at least some modifications in content or structure be made.

PURPOSE AND USES

The purposes of theory derivation are to acquire a means of explanation and prediction about some phenomenon that is currently poorly understood, or for which there is no present means to study it, or for which there is no theory at all. Theory derivation is particularly useful where no data are available or where new insights about a phenomenon are needed to inspire research and testing. Theory derivation is useful when a theorist has a set of concepts that are somehow related to each other, but has no structural way to represent those relationships. (See Chapter 8 for more detailed description of structure derivation.) In this case, the theorist might find that some other field of interest has a structure in one of its theories that is analogous to the relationships of the concepts in which he or she is interested. The theorist may use the derivation strategy appropriately by adopting and adapting the structure to fit the concepts being considered. This adds to the body of knowledge in the theorist's field in a significant and rapid way that might not have happened for some time without the derivation strategy. An example of this is Nierenberg's use of Maslow's hierarchical structure of needs to derive a theory of negotiation (1968; 1973).

Theory derivation is also very useful when a theorist has some ideas about the basic structure of a phenomenon but has no concepts to describe it. Another theory in a different field may provide the theorist with a set of analogous concepts that can help describe the phenomenon if modified slightly. Again, this procedure rapidly adds to the body of knowledge in the theorist's own field. One example of this strategy is one we used in Chapter 5, where Roy (1976) developed the concepts of focal, contextual, and residual stimuli in patient assessment from a psychophysics theory by Helson.

Several examples of theory derivation come quickly to mind when we consider systems theory. Many of our nursing models in their original form have been direct derivations from systems theory—Roy (1976), Neuman (1980), and others have significant aspects of theory derivation strategies in them.

PROCEDURES FOR THEORY DERIVATION

Theory derivation can be discussed as a series of sequential steps. The actual process may not occur sequentially. Many times theory derivation becomes an iterative process. That is, the theorist repeats some or all of the steps until the level of sophistication of the theory is acceptable.

There are several basic steps in theory derivation:

1. Become thoroughly familiar with the literature on the topic of interest. This implies that the theorist is cognizant of the level of theory development in his or her field and has evaluated the scientific usefulness of any such developments. If none of the current theories are suitable for the purpose of the theorist then theory derivation can proceed.

2. Read widely in other fields for ideas. Reading widely enables a theorist to understand ways of putting theory together in other disciplines. Reading widely is not enough. The theorist must read while allowing imagination and creativity free reign. Discovering analogies is often done accidentally or as a creative intuitive leap rather than systematically.

3. Select a parent theory to use for derivation. The parent theory should be chosen because it offers a new and insightful way of explaining or predicting about a phenomenon in the theorist's field of interest. Just any theory won't do. Many theories will shed no light at all on the concepts of interest or will provide no useful structure

for the concepts and are therefore worthless to the theorist. Keep in mind here that the whole parent theory may not be needed to form the new theory. Only those portions that are analogous and therefore relevant need be used.

4. Identify what content and/or structure from the parent theory is to be used. Perhaps only the concepts or only the statements are analogous, but not the structure. Or perhaps the structure is perfect but the parent concepts and statements are not. Perhaps the theorist needs both concepts and statements as well as structure. In the derivation strategy, the theorist is free to choose what best fits the needs of the situation.

5. Develop or redefine any new concepts or statements from the content or structure of the parent theory in terms of the phenomenon of interest to the theorist. This is the hardest part of theory derivation, but also the most fun. It requires creativity and thoughtfulness on the part of the theorist. Basically, the concepts or structure that is borrowed from the parent field is modified in such a way that it becomes meaningful in the theorist's field. Often the modifications are small, but occasionally they will need to be substantial before the theory makes sense in the new setting.

Cronkite and Moos *Propositions*	*Wewers and Lenz* *Derivations*
1. Pretreatment symptoms such as alcohol consumption, type of drinker, depression, and occupational functioning are related to alcohol treatment outcomes (p. 48).	1. Pretreatment symptoms such as cigarette consumption and type of smoker are related to smoking relapse (p. 48).
2. "Stressful life events were negatively associated with some aspects of recovery" (p. 49).	2. "Both the social contextual stressor of major life events and the internal stressor of craving" are associated with smoking relapse (p. 49).
3. Family environment is "weakly related to alcohol recovery" (p. 49).	3. "Long term smoking cessation is associated with having family members who are nonsmokers or who had previously been able to quit smoking" (p. 49).

We are giving you several brief examples of theory derivation. Often, an example is clearer than an explanation alone can be. Let us begin with Wewers and Lenz's (1987) theory of relapse among ex-smokers that they derived from Cronkite and Moos's theory of post-treatment functioning of alcoholics (1980). Wewers and Lenz primarily used content derivation but also derived a simplified structure. Listed on page 186 are three propositions from Cronkite and Moos with the derivations made by Wewers and Lenz. In some cases we have adapted the wording of the propositions to show the derivations more clearly.

Because there was a rich literature already available on smoking, Wewers and Lenz adopted propositions in their derivation that fit knowledge specifically about smoking. This is an excellent example of how to use the strategy flexibly in theory-building efforts.

Another example in which theorists used a derivation strategy is one in which Maccia and Maccia used both concepts and structure of a theory of eye blinks to derive a theory of education. Listed below are a few of the principles and their derivations from Maccia and Maccia's work (Maccia & Maccia, 1963).

Parent Theory	*Maccia et al.*
1. Either the eyes are or are not covered by lids.	1. Either the student is distracted or attentive.
2. Blinking functions to protect the eyes from contact and to rest the retina and the ocular muscles.	2. Distraction functions to protect the student from mental stress and to rest from mental effort.
3. Blinking may be either reflexive or nonreflexive.	3. Distraction may be either voluntary or nonvoluntary.
4. Reflex blinking may be inhibited by a fixation object or by drugs.	4. Nonvoluntary distraction may be inhibited by attention cues or by drugs.
5. Nonreflexive blinking may occur if seeing is un-wanted.	5. Voluntary distraction may occur if learning is un-wanted.

As you can see, theory derivation can happen using two widely disparate fields. It is the theorist's creativity and intuition that provide the insight into the analogy.

Now that we have seen two examples in which both concepts and structure were used in theory derivation, let us examine one example in which only concepts were used and another example in which only structure was used.

The example we would like to use of a theory derivation where the concepts from the parent theory were used, but not the structure, is one by Suchman on predicting health behavior. Using the traditional epidemiological concepts of "host," "agent," and "environment," Suchman modified these concepts to become "personal readiness," "situational factors," and "social control factors," respectively. In his studies to test his new concepts, personal readiness factors were found to be the most predictive of the adoption of a health protection measure. Social control and situational factors were much less predictive of adoption of a health protection measure (Suchman, 1967).

An example in which the structure, but not the concepts, was derived into a new theory is Lawrence Kohlberg's theory of moral development, which he based on the structure of Piaget's theory of cognitive development. Both theories speak to the relationship of the child's age to its cognitive or moral development. Below we have listed both Piaget's structure and the derivation from it made by Kohlberg (Piaget, 1950; Piaget and Inhelder, 1958; Kohlberg, 1964).

Piaget	Kohlberg
Level I: Preoperational Phase	Level I: Premoral Level
1. Sensorimotor stage	Type 1: Punishment and obedience orientation
2. Preconceptual stage	Type 2: Naive instrumental hedonism
Level II: Concrete Operations Phase	Level II: Morality of Conventional Role-Conformity
1. Intuitive state	Type 3: Good boy morality
2. Concrete operation state	Type 4: Authority maintaining morality
Level III: Formal Operations Phase	Level III: Morality of Self-Accepted Moral Principles
1. Formal operations state	Type 5: Morality of control, individual rights, and democratically accepted law
	Type 6: Morality of individual principles of conscience

Kohlberg used the phase/stage structure of Piaget's levels of cognitive development and modified it to organize his concepts of the levels of moral reasoning. This strategy helped him to make clear the orderliness of moral development and, in addition, saved him a considerable amount of development time. In this case, the parent field was not so disparate from Kohlberg's as was the eye blink theory from that of Maccia and Maccia. But in both cases, the discovery of the analogous relationships between the parent theory and the new theory was extremely helpful to the theorist by facilitating the construction efforts.

Derived theories, it must be remembered, are constructed in the context of discovery. The theories thus developed have no validity until they are subjected to empirical testing in the context of justification. Even if the theory is extremely relevant to practice or research, it must first be validated before it can be used.

Several methods that may be used to test theories, for example, experimental designs for groups or single subjects and *ex post facto* designs, are presented in Chapter 7. In addition, Chapter 9 on theory analysis or Chapter 12 on theory testing may also be useful. Even though these methods are presented here as developmental strategies, they may be modified easily for use in theory testing. Additional help may be found in the research references included here and in several other chapters.

Another way to test theory is to subject it to examination in light of the existing literature on the topic. Is there any support in the literature that makes it more plausible or likely? Finally, if the theory is reliable in predicting outcomes, this reliability provides an additional measure of support. None of these methods can substitute for a full-scale empirical test, but they can provide a general estimate of the theory's plausibility.

ADVANTAGES AND LIMITATIONS

The major advantage of theory derivation is that it is a reasonably easy and quick way to obtain formal theory in new areas of interest. It is an exciting exercise in that it requires the theorist to use creativity and imagination in seeing analogies from one field and modifying them for use in a new field. In addition, theory derivation provides a way of arriving at explanation and prediction about a phenomenon where there may be little or no information, literature, or formal studies.

The major disadvantage of theory derivation is that novice theorists become so excited about their new generalizations that they fail to take into account any dissimilarities, or dis-analogies, present in the parent theory. These dis-analogies should at least be considered for any valuable information that they might provide in the "new" theory.

A second disadvantage is that the theorist must be familiar with a number of fields of interest other than his or her own. This implies reading widely and being constantly on the alert for new and profitable analogies. In addition, the theorist must be thoroughly familiar with the literature and current thinking about his or her particular area of interest. Otherwise, when the time comes to draw an analogy, the theorist will have difficulty choosing appropriate boundaries for the new theory.

UTILIZING THE RESULTS OF THEORY DERIVATION

We have said the uses of theory derivation are to provide structure when only concepts are available, to provide concepts when only structure is available, or to provide both concepts and structure as an efficient way to begin theory development. The results of theory derivation are easily used in nursing education, practice, research, and theory development.

In education, theory derivation is an excellent way to obtain a theoretical framework for curriculum building. In addition, it can be used as a teaching tool with graduate students as a way to introduce them to theorizing in general.

Theory derivation can provide significant new insights for clinical practice. Clinicians can provide themselves with a useful theoretical framework to guide their practice by using the results of theory derivation.

In research and theory development, theory derivation is a simple way to design a research program. Moving concepts and/or structure from the parent field with appropriate changes yields a rich source of potential hypotheses for study, as Wewers and Lenz demonstrated. It is a very efficient strategy for achieving a body of knowledge about a phenomenon.

SUMMARY

Theory derivation is the process of using analogy to obtain explanations or predictions about a phenomenon in one field from explanations or predictions in another field. Theory derivation is an excellent way of obtaining rapid theory development in the new field. Both concepts and structure can be moved from the parent field to the new one undergoing modifications along the way.

There are five steps to theory derivation: (1) become thoroughly familiar with the topic of interest; (2) read widely in other fields, allowing your imagination to help you find useful analogies; (3) select a parent theory to use for derivation; (4) identify what content and/or structure from the parent theory is to be used; (5) modify or redefine new concepts and/or statements in terms of the phenomenon of interest.

Once the new theory has been formulated, it must be tested empirically to validate that the new concepts and structure actually reflect reality in the new field.

The advantages of theory derivation are the ease and rapidity with which new constructions can be made. One disadvantage is that the theorist must be widely read in several fields as well as his or her own field. In addition, the theorist must remember to consider the dissimilarities as well as the similarities between the parent field and the new field.

Theory derivation is a highly workable strategy for nursing at this point in our development of a knowledge base. It provides a means of rapid acquisition of theory with meaningful content. If carefully done and carefully tested, derived theories could play an immediate role in the development of scientific knowledge in nursing.

PRACTICE EXERCISES

Below is a list of 17 relational statements from a general systems theory for behavioral science (Miller, 1955). Using the derivation strategy in this chapter, construct a new theory for nursing in your own particular area of clinical interest. You don't have to include all 17 statements. Choose the ones most relevant to your area of interest. Remember that an open system is one that is bounded in space and time and that exchanges energy and information with its subsystems and with its environment (suprasystem).

A. Greater energy is required for transmission across a boundary than for transmission within the environment or within a subsystem.

B. Spread of energy or information throughout systems is quantitatively comparable.

C. There is a constant systematic distortion—or alteration—between inputs of energy or information into the system and outputs from the system.

D. The distortion of a system is the sum of the effects of processes that subtract from the input to reduce the strains in subsystems or add to the output to reduce the strains.

E. When variables in a system return to equilibrium after stress, the rate of return and the strength of the restorative forces are stronger than a linear function of the amount of displacement from the equilibrium point.

F. Living systems respond to continuously increasing stress first by a lag in response, then by overcompensation, then by collapse of the system.

G. Systems that survive employ the least expensive defenses against stress first and increasingly more expensive ones later.

H. Systems that survive perform at an optimum efficiency for maximum power output, which is always less than maximum efficiency.

I. When a system's negative feedback discontinues, its steady state vanishes, its boundaries disappear, and the system ends.

J. The output of a system is always less than its input.

K. Decentralization of the maintenance of variables in equilibrium is always more expensive of energy than centralization although it may increase utility.

L. As decentralization increases, subsystems increasingly act without the benefit of information available elsewhere in the system.

M. The more subsystems there are in efficient systems, the more variables they can maintain in equilibrium.

N. The more subsystems there are in efficient systems, the more subsystems whose destruction will cause the system to collapse.

O. When reduction of several strains is not possible simultaneously, the order in which they are reduced in systems that survive is from strongest to weakest, if the effort required for reduction is the same.

P. Up to a maximum, the more energy in a system devoted to information processing, the more likely the system is to survive.

Q. When one living species feeds on another in a given suprasystem, and both species continue to survive, an oscillation of numbers of predators and prey occurs around an equilibrium point.[1]

Just for fun, we derived a theory about graduate students in nursing. You may wish to compare your theory with ours below. We chose to use only a few statements to give you an example of how

[1]From Miller JG: Toward a general theory for behavioral science. Amer Psychol 10:9, 513–531, 1955. Copyright (1955) by the American Psychological Association. Reprinted by permission of the publisher and the author.

derivation might work. We have used the same alphabetical notation as the parent theory statements to help you identify where our statements come from.

A. Graduate students in nursing communicate with each other more efficiently than with their professors.
C. When graduate students are told the course requirements at the beginning of a course, they will ask for clarification of those requirements before mid-term.
F. 1. The nearer exams or deadlines approach, the more study groups are formed.
   2. As exams or deadlines approach, the illness rate in students increases.
O. When several projects are due at once, graduate students will complete the most difficult project first.
P. The more reading and thinking done by the student, the more likely he or she is to complete the degree.
J. Graduate students must complete a full curriculum in order to have enough skills to complete a thesis or dissertation.
I. When the final thesis or dissertation defense is completed, the student graduates.

REFERENCES

Cronkite RC, Moos RH: Determinants of the post-treatment functioning of alcoholic patients: A conceptual framework. J Consult Clin Psychol 48: 305–316, 1980.

Kohlberg L: Development of moral character and moral ideology. In (M Hoffman & L Hoffman, eds.), Review of Child Development Research. New York: Russell Sage Foundation, 1964, 383–431.

Maccia ES, Maccia GS, Jewett RE: Construction of Educational Theory Models. Cooperative Research Project #1632. Columbus, Ohio: Ohio State Univ. Research Foundation, 1963.

Miller JG: Toward a general theory for behavioral science. Amer Psychol 10:9: 513–531, 1955.

Nierenberg GI: The Art of Negotiating. New York: Hawthorne, 1968.

Nierenberg GI: Fundamentals of Negotiating. New York: Hawthorne, 1973.

Neuman B: The Betty Neuman health care systems model: A total person approach to patient problems. In (JP Riehl & C Roy, eds.), Conceptual Models for Nursing Practice. 2d ed. New York: Appleton-Century-Crofts, 1980.

Piaget J: The Psychology of Intelligence. London: Routledge and Kegan Paul, 1950.

Piaget J, Inhelder B: The Growth of Logical Thinking from Childhood to Adolescence. New York: Basic Books, 1958.

Rogers ME: An Introduction to the Theoretical Basis of Nursing. Philadelphia: F.A. Davis, 1970.

Roy C: Introduction to Nursing: An Adaptation Model. Englewood Cliffs, N.J.: Prentice-Hall, 1976.

Suchman EA: Preventive health behavior: A model for research on community health campaigns. J Health Social Behav 8:197, 1967.
Wewers ME, Lenz E: Relapse among ex-smokers: An example of theory
derivation. Adv Nurs Sci 9(2): 44–53, 1987.

ADDITIONAL READINGS

Burr JW: Theory Construction in Sociology of the Family. New York: John
Wiley, 1973.
Ghiselin B (ed.): The Creative Process: A Symposium. New York: New Amer-
ican Library, 1952.
Kaplan A: The Conduct of Inquiry. New York: Chandler, 1964.
Miller JG: Living Systems. New York: McGraw-hill, 1978.
Olson RW: The Art of Creative Thinking: A Practical Guide. New York:
Barnes and Noble Books, 1980.

PART V

Perspectives on Nursing Science

In this final part of the book, we step back and try to get the long view. Our goal is to put the specifics of theory development into context. First, Chapter 12 focuses on the step after theory development: theory testing. This is an important and often neglected activity in evolving the theoretical basis for the nursing discipline. Theory testing involves both logical operations and empirical research, both of which are briefly addressed in Chapter 12. Next, to get an idea about emerging foci of nursing theory, the content of recent nursing research reports is analyzed and presented. These content foci are seen as specific elaborations of the metaparadigm concepts of person, environment, health, and nursing. Four emerging foci for nursing theory are identified: (1) health behaviors and/or health status; (2) stress and coping; (3) transitions; and (4) person–environment interactions. In considering these foci, the level of theory development most likely to have a direct impact on practice is addressed. A proposal is offered for how theoretical nursing can be more closely related to the practice of nursing.

While the bulk of this book has necessarily been directed to the scientific dimensions of nursing, alternative sources of knowledge and ways of knowing are of concern when nursing is viewed from a more comprehensive perspective. Thus, in Chapter 13 we provide a review of alternate sources of knowledge and the place of scientific theory development in relation to them. Finally, we suggest that the use of multiple perspectives in knowledge development is most appropriate.

195

12

Theory Refinement: Testing and Emerging Theoretical Foci

INTRODUCTION

The success of this book will be measured more by the conceptual and theoretical work it generates than by anything we say. This being so, we would like to focus on two topics closely related to theory development strategies: theory testing and the substantive foci of theory that we see on the horizon. Important work is occurring in nursing on both these fronts.

THEORY TESTING

In Chapter 2, we presented a model of the phases in the development of nursing science (see Figure 2.2). The nine chapters preceding this one have been devoted to the first phases depicted in the model: developing concepts, statements, and theories in nursing. Theory testing is a vital next phase that follows the initial development of theory. Indeed, the sequential phases of development, testing, revision, and retesting of theory portrayed in our model demonstrate the necessary and reciprocal links between the contexts of discovery and justification in building nursing science. In this line, Marx (1963) has said:

> We need to recognize most explicitly that *both* discovery *and* confirmation are necessary to effective scientific work. The most

ingenious theories are limited (sic) value until empirical tests are
produced; the best confirmed proposition is of little value unless
it deals with meaningful variables (p. 13).

Unfortunately, the struggle to develop theory in nursing has often
left the testing of theory neglected.

Further, assessing the empirical validity of a theory is hampered
by lack of clarity about what constitutes sound theory-testing research. In this line Silva (1986) has proposed seven evaluation criteria that studies aimed at testing conceptual models (grand theories)
should ideally meet. Her work is particularly important because it
provides methodological reference points that have been missing
from most previous literature on theory testing. Thus, our understanding of what constitutes adequate theory testing has been sharp-
ened by her work. Because the concern in this section is with testing
a wide variety of middle-range theories that may inform us about
nursing phenomena, we propose an adaptation of Silva's criteria to
fit this more specific application:

1. The purpose of the study is to determine the empirical validity of
   a designated theory's assumptions or propositions (internal theoretical statements).
2. The theory is explicitly stated as the rationale for the research.
3. The theory's internal structure (key propositions and their interrelationships) is explicitly stated so that its relationship to study
   hypotheses is clear.
4. The study hypotheses are clearly deduced from the theory's assumptions or propositions.
5. The study hypotheses are empirically tested in an appropriate
   research design using sound and relevant instruments and suitable study participants.
6. As a result of the empirical testing, evidence exists of the validity
   or invalidity of the designated assumptions or propositions of the
   theory.
7. This evidence is considered specifically as it supports, refutes, or
   explains relevant aspects of the theory.

However, even these criteria are lacking in one regard. Consider
that it is conceivable that one could derive hypotheses from a theory
that were compatible with it as well as several other theories and,
additionally, that the hypotheses were consistently shown to be congruent with empirical observations. For example, the hypothesis that
the poor will experience more health problems than the wealthy is
compatible with several theoretical models. Similarly, predicting on
theoretical grounds that patients receiving individualized nursing

intervention will demonstrate more skill in self care than those receiving routine care may well be derivable from a number of theories. Further, testing a hypothesis such as either of the above carries a low risk for any theories from which they are derived because they would be expected to be supported by the data. Indeed both of the examples given are vague hypotheses that would be difficult to reject. Thus, theory testing is more complex than simply deriving hypotheses and testing them. Not only must researchers be able to derive hypotheses, but they should do so in a way that puts a theory at high risk for falsification (Popper, 1965). To be falsifiable, a theory must be able to predict with enough specificity that empirical results that are incompatible with the theory can be derived clearly (Fawcett & Downs, 1986, pp. 59–61). Wallace (1971) presented an example of this principle in operation.

> For a simple example, the hypothesis that "all human groups are either stratified or not stratified" is untestable in principle because it does not rule out any logically possible empirical findings. The hypothesis that "all human groups are stratified," however, is testable because it asserts that the discovery of an unstratified human group, though logically possible, will not in fact occur (p. 78).

To repeat an old saw: a theory that predicts everything predicts nothing. Or, in the words of Popper, "Every 'good' scientific theory is a prohibition: it forbids certain things to happen. The more a theory forbids, the better it is" (1965, p. 36). Thus, we add still another criterion for theory testing:

8. The hypotheses used to test a specific theory are designed to put the theory at risk for falsification by virtue of their specificity and compatibility with only a limited set of events.

According to this last criterion, the more specific the predictions that can be made from a theory, the more readily it can be falsified and the narrower the range of data that will support the theory. In testing theories, one must judge how well the results of testing fit with the theories. As theoretical predictions increase in precision, the judgment about "fit" becomes less ambiguous and less arbitrary (Blalock, 1979). Further, if the results of testing highly specific hypotheses result in data that are very consistent with predictions, the theory is judged to be both falsifiable and empirically valid. Consider the following examples. The prediction that "A is associated with B" is less specific than the prediction that "in every case of B, it is preceded by the occurrence of A." Still more precise is the hypothesis that "B will reach a critical value of 75 units only if A reaches a level of 50 units or more." As hypotheses formulated in nursing research move increasingly from the former type to the latter, the falisifiability of theories will increase.

Unfortunately, empirical validity (correspondence of a theory with empirical evidence) is not an absolute quality of theories; it is tied to the existing evidence pertinent to the theory. As further research is done, a theory that was judged empirically valid at one time may be considered less valid at a later time. Thus, as additional tests of a theory provide evidence that is compatible or incompatible with theoretical predictions, empirical validity grows or shrinks respectively.

Theory testing is complicated by still another dimension, assumptions made in designing testing conditions (Hempel, 1966, pp. 19–32). These assumptions include a wide range of explicit and implicit beliefs such as (1) adequate reliability and validity of measurement procedures used, (2) absence of contaminating circumstances during data collection, and (3) accuracy of any scientific "facts" assumed to be true in designing the research procedures. Where results support a theory, one erroneously may have discounted an alternate explanation of the results. Where results do not support a theoretical prediction, an error may lie not in the theory itself but in the testing conditions. Thus, no one test will definitively refute or substantiate a theory. Theory testing is rather the weight of *accumulated* testing results in varied researches. Replication of research that tests a promising theory is consequently a strategic aspect in building nursing science.

A final problem in theory testing rests in the theorist and researcher. It is often easier to cling to a familiar and cherished theory than to abandon it. Surely theorists and researchers are human too! While "facts" may seem irrefutable, their interpretation may certainly be influenced by subjective factors. For this reason, we advocate that theory testing be executed using, where possible, multiple competing hypotheses (Platt, 1964). To do this requires that a researcher derive research hypotheses about a phenomenon from several theories and design research to test concurrently each of these. Simultaneously proposing and testing several competing theoretically based hypotheses for their fit and scientific utility reduces the danger that a researcher will be overly wedded to any one theory. Proposing hypotheses from several competing theories and then simultaneously testing these has the added advantage of accelerating the scientific process. Rather than testing one theory, finding it equivocal, and then moving on to testing another, this entire sequence can be merged into one research effort. In actual practice, this approach has been useful in evaluating competing theoretical models of mother-infant relationships (Walker, 1984).

As we pointed out in the initial chapter of this book, nursing has generated theory at many levels. Only theory that is sufficiently refined and proposes measurable models of reality, however, is amenable to rigorous testing. Well-articulated theories decrease the arbitrariness of judgments about their merits. This is especially important if a theory base is used in defining directions for policy and practice. Testability of a theory and its empirical validity are of equal or greater importance in nursing as a practice discipline than to basic sciences. The public trust in a profession warrants using the very best procedures in making scientific judgments that have social import.

EMERGING THEORETICAL FOCI IN NURSING

Identification of the metaparadigm concepts of person, health, environment, and nursing have signaled an area of consensus within nursing (Fawcett, 1984). Still these concepts represent the perspectives of nursing at a very abstract level without interrelationships among the concepts being specified. To sharpen the focus of the metaparadigm concepts as they relate specifically to nursing, several writers have proposed that a distinctive nursing concern involves the interrelatedness of the metaparadigm concepts (Newman, 1983; Chick & Meleis, 1986; Clarke & Driever, 1983). Further, additional concepts may be needed to express the specific nursing concern embodied in the interrelationship of person, health, environment, and nursing. In this regard Clarke and Driever (1983) have proposed a nursing construct of vulnerability, and Chick & Meleis (1986) have offered the concept of transitions as specific elaborations of the interrelatedness of the metaparadigm concepts.

In an effort to further capture what may be emerging nursing elaborations of the metaparadigm concepts, we conducted an informal content analysis to determine thematic foci present within present-day nursing literature. (Specific theories identified during the analysis are reported in Chapter 1. However, in most articles the theoretical bases for studies were not well defined. Thus we reanalyzed each article for its thematic focus. Themes were extrapolated from titles, aims, and methods.) The literature used for this analysis was six recent issues from each of two nursing research journals, *Nursing Research* and *Research in Nursing and Health*. These journals were selected because they were not limited to one clinical specialty or a specific topical focus and because we believed that research journals would be the medium in which nursing elaborations of metaparadigm concepts would be most explicitly expressed.

TABLE 12.1. EMERGING CONCEPTUAL FOCI IN NURSING RESEARCH[a]

Title	Author(s)/date
Focus 1 Health Behavior and Health Status	
Attitudes, Subjective Norms, and Intentions to Engage in Health Behaviors	Pender & Pender, 1986
Theoretical Model Testing to Identify Personality Variables Effecting Preventive Behaviors	Murdaugh & Hinshaw, 1986
Relationship of Demographic, Life-style, and Stress Variables to Blood Pressure in Adolescents	Thomas & Groer, 1986
Normal and Overweight Adults: Perceived Weight and Health Behavior Characteristics	Laffrey, 1986
Use of the Health Belief Model in Determining Frequency of Breast Self-Examination	Champion, 1985
Mothers' Health Beliefs and Use of Well-Baby Services Among a High-Risk Population	Kviz, Dawkins, & Ervin, 1985
The Relationship of Movement and Time to Older Adults' Functional Health	Engle, 1986
Focus 2 Stress and Coping	
Parent Coping, A Replication	Ventura, 1986
Human Responses to Chronic Illness: Physiologic and Psychosocial Adaptation	Pollock, 1986
Stressors Associated with Coronary Bypass Surgery	Carr & Powers, 1986
Effect of Preoperative Instruction on Postoperative Outcomes: A Meta-Analysis	Hathaway, 1986
Effects of Cognitive and Pharmacologic Strategies on Analogued Labor Pain	Geden, Beck, Anderson, Kennish, & Mueller-Heinze, 1986
Perceived Job Stress, Job Satisfaction, and Psychological Symptoms in Critical Care Nursing	Norbeck, 1985
Stress, Coping Behaviors, and Recommendations for Intensive Care and Medical Surgical Ward Registered Nurses	Kelly & Cross, 1985

[a]*Note:* While titles are listed here, classification of articles was based on study aims and methods, not solely titles. Articles cited here may be found in *Nursing Research* 35 and *Research in Nursing and Health* 8, Issues 2–4, and 9, Issues 1–3.

Title	Author(s)/date
Focus 3 Developmental and Health-Related Transitions	
Role Conflict, Marital Satisfaction, Employment Role Attitude, and Transition to the Maternal Role	Majewski, 1986
Social Support, Stress, and Health: A Comparison of Expectant Mothers and Fathers	Brown, 1986
Measure of Attitude Toward Menopause Using the Semantic Differential Model	Bowles, 1986
Developmental Progress in Very Low Birth Weight Infants During the First Year of Life	Schraeder, 1986
Effect of Role Clarity and Empathy on Support Role Performance and Anxiety	Bramwell & Whall, 1986
Developmental Resources and Depression in the Elderly	Reed, 1986
The Relationship of Developmental Variables to Maternal Behavior	Mercer, 1986
Focus 4 Person–Environment Interactions	
Arthritis Patients' Self-Reported Affective States and Their Caregivers' Perceptions	Muhlenkamp & Joyner, 1986
Temperament in Very Low Birth Weight Infants	Medoff-Cooper, 1986
Father-Infant Interaction: Effects of Social Competence and Infant State	Jones & Lenz, 1986
Nurse Practitioner-Patient Interactional Analyses During Well Child Visits	Webster-Stratton, Glascock, & McCarthy, 1986
Initial Handling of Newborn Infants by Vaginally and Cesarian-Delivered Mothers	Tulman, 1986
Hypertension, Perceived Clinician Empathy, and Patient Self-Disclosure	Dawson, 1985
Environmental Support for Autonomy in the Institutionalized Elderly	Ryden, 1985

Using a concept synthesis process, the content of each article was identified in terms of the primary phenomenon on which it focused (in title, aims, and methods). From this, higher-order categories were iteratively developed. We found that roughly 60 percent of the 123 articles that we examined focused on the description, the explanation, the prediction, or the control of one or more of the following phenomena:

1. Health behavior and/or health status (health behavior practices and/or physical and mental health–illness levels)
2. Stress and coping (sources of stress and responses to manage stress)
3. Transitions related to developmental change or illness (changes in pattern of functioning or role related to developmental processes or illness)
4. Person–environment interactions (influence of the interpersonal and social environment on the person and vice versa)

Each of these four theoretical foci occurred among diverse populations of clients suggesting that these do not represent traditional clinical areas (see Table 12.1 on pp. 202–203 for samples of articles in each category).

While we cannot predict the theoretical foci that will be most promising for nursing's future development, each of these support the contention that theorizing that elaborates the interrelatedness among metaparadigm concepts is needed. Further, each could serve as the focal point for development and testing of specific middle-range theories about nursing phenomena. As illustrated in Figure 1.1 in Chapter 1, grand theories may guide the development of middle-range theories. These in turn may serve to further refine concepts and relationships proposed at the grand theory level as well as direct the development of theory at the practice level in the form of theory-based interventions.

Let us illustrate how elaborations of the metaparadigm concepts may promote growth of theory at more than one level. One of the emerging foci, that of transitions, has been the object of careful analysis by Chick and Meleis (1986), who demonstrated its link to metaparadigm concepts. Additionally, they proposed that transitions are related to shifts in self-care capacities (p. 244), that is, potential changes in health behaviors, a middle-range proposition. In relating the concept of transitions to the practice level, they proposed that the dimensions of time, pattern, type of transition, and timing of intervention be considered (pp. 244–245). In a related vein Barnard (1982) has proposed that a central concern of nursing is monitoring of transitional stages (p. 6). Thus, middle-range concepts that serve to elaborate the metaparadigm concepts but also go beyond them in degree of specificity may add to the development of theory at more than one level.

Ultimately, practice informed by well-developed middle-range theories could span the gap that currently exists between grand theories and the specific phenomena of nursing practice. In this line Murphy and Hoeffer (1983) have argued that a hiatus has developed between specialty areas of practice and nursing theory development, especially at the level of the metaparadigm concepts of person, environment, health, and nursing. While the theory-practice gap is often approached as a failure of some institutional process, we argue that the nature of extant nursing theory itself is at least partially at fault and hence has contributed to the gap.

Murphy and Hoeffer have identified three trends that have led to slippage in the role that nursing specialties have played in nursing theory development:

1. Defining nursing as a discipline separate from medicine
2. Educating entry-level generalists
3. Developing conceptual frameworks (1983, p. 32)

They note that the third trend has led to widespread use of conceptual models (what we have termed "grand theories"), yet none of these has delineated the role of specialties in theory development. They then propose that "nursing specialties can best contribute to nursing science by generating middle-range or limited-scope theories" (1983, pp. 34–35). It is the latter level of theory that they see as more directly relevant to practice concerns compared to grand theory.

We concur with the thrust of Murphy and Hoeffer's position, but would add that its force applies not only to specialty practice but to all realms of nursing practice. Grand theories have served an invaluable role in delineating what constitutes a distinctively nursing point of view. Now middle-range theories are urgently needed to mediate between grand theories and specific phenomena encountered at the level of practice.

CONCLUSION

Advances in thinking about both testing of theories and emerging theoretical foci suggest that nursing theory development and nursing research are becoming more closely linked. Theorizing and research are thought of less and less as two independent acts. As more well-formed middle-range theories are developed, the link between a study's theory base and its hypotheses, design, instrumentation, and data analysis will be strengthened.

Close interdependence between theory and research is essential if nursing is to build a sound body of knowledge for practice. Bold new theories are needed to vitalize research programs. In turn, focused, well-designed research is needed to challenge and refine nursing theory. Progress on each of these fronts is increasingly evident in nursing publications. Indeed nursing may well be on the verge of a knowledge revolution because of these forces.

REFERENCES

Barnard KE: The research cycle: Nursing, the profession, the discipline. Proceedings of the 1982 Conference of the Western Society for Research in Nursing. Western Journal of Nursing Research 4(3): 1–12, 1982.

Blalock HM: Dilemmas and strategies of theory construction. In (WE Snizek, ER Fuhrman, & MK Miller, eds.), Contemporary Issues in Theory and Research: A Metasociological Perspective. Westport, Conn.: Greenwood Press, 1979.

Chick N, Meleis AI: Transitions: A nursing concern. In (PL Chinn, ed.), Nursing Research Methodology. Rockville, Md.: Aspen, 1986.

Clarke HF, Driever MJ: Vulnerability: The development of a construct for nursing. In (PL Chinn, ed.), Advances in Nursing Theory Development. Rockville, Md.: Aspen, 1983.

Fawcett J: The metaparadigm of nursing: Present status and future refinements. Image 16: 84–87, 1984.

Fawcett J, Downs FS: The Relationship of Theory and Research. Norwalk, Conn.: Appleton-Century-Crofts, 1986.

Hempel CG: Philosophy of Natural Science. Englewood Cliffs, N.J.: Prentice-Hall, 1966.

Marx MH: The general nature of theory construction. In (MH Marx, ed.), Theories in Contemporary Psychology. New York: Macmillan, 1963.

Murphy SA, Hoeffer B: Role of the specialties in nursing science. Adv Nurs Sci 5(4): 31–39, 1983.

Newman MA: The continuing revolution: A history of nursing science. In (NL Chaska, ed.), The Nursing Profession: A Time to Speak. New York: McGraw-Hill, 1983.

Platt JR: Strong inference. Science 146: 347–352, 1964.

Popper KR: Conjectures and Refutations. New York: Basic Books, 1965.

Silva MC: Research testing nursing theory: State of the art. Adv Nurs Sci 9(1): 1–11, 1986.

Walker LO: Strategy for theory development: Deductive approach. Proceedings of the First Nursing Science Colloquium. Boston: Boston University School of Nursing, 1984, 17–35.

Wallace WL: The Logic of Science in Sociology. New York: Aldine, 1971.

ADDITIONAL READINGS

Readings on Theory Testing

Blalock HM: Dilemmas and strategies of theory construction. In (WE Snizek, ER Fuhrman, & MK Miller, eds.), Contemporary Issues in Theory and Research: A Metasociological Perspective. Westport, Conn.: Greenwood Press, 1979.

Field M: Causal inference in behavioral research. Adv Nurs Sci 2(1): 81–93, 1979.

Gibbs JP: Part 3. Test of theories. Sociological Theory Construction. Hinsdale, Ill.: Dryden Press, 1972.

Hinshaw AS: Theoretical model testing: Full utilization of data. Western Journal of Nursing Research 6: 5–9, 1984.

Jacobs MK: Can nursing theory be tested? In (PL Chinn, ed.), Nursing Research Methodology. Rockville, Md.: Aspen, 1986.

Kerlinger FN, Pedhazur EJ: Chapter 17. Theory, application, and multiple regression in behavioral research. In Multiple Regression in Behavioral Research. New York: Holt, Rinehart & Winston, 1973.

Mullins NC: Chapter 6. Empirical testing. In The Art of Theory: Construction and Use. New York: Harper & Row, 1971.

Munro BH: Dropouts from nursing education: Path analysis of a national sample. Nurs Res 29: 371–377, 1980.

Popper KR: Conjectures and Refutations. New York: Basic Books, 1962.

Reynolds BD: Chapter 6. Testing theories. In A Primer in Theory Construction. Indianapolis: Bobbs-Merrill, 1971.

Schwirian PM: Toward an explanatory model of nursing performance. Nurs Res 30: 247–253, 1981.

Wallace WL: Chapter 5. Tests of hypotheses; decisions to accept or reject hypotheses; logical inference; theories. In The Logic of Science of Sociology. New York: Aldine, 1971.

Zetterberg HL: On Theory and Verification in Sociology. Totowa, N.J.: Bedminster Press, 1965.

13

Dimensions of Nursing Knowledge

INTRODUCTION

In this final chapter we take yet another step back to gain an even broader view by focusing on the dimensions of knowledge in nursing. In order to do this, we must first make clear the distinctions between knowing, knowledge itself, knowledge generation, and knowledge refinement.

To know is to "be cognizant, conscious or aware of, to perceive or comprehend with clearness and certainty" (Halsey, 1979). Knowing is a personal, internal experience of cognition. Knowing something may or may not involve understanding what is known. Understanding involves knowing not just facts but having an insight into the meaning, significance, and implications of those facts (Halsey, 1979).

Knowledge is "familiarity, understanding, awareness, or information acquired through experience, study, or observation; the sum or range of that which is or can be perceived or learned" (Halsey, 1979). Knowledge then is the product of knowing. It is experiential and summative.

To generate is to produce, cause to be, or bring into existence (Halsey, 1979). So knowledge generation is to produce or bring into existence information, awareness, or understanding through experience, study, or observation.

To refine is "to reduce to a pure state; to make improvement by introducing subtleties or distinctions" (Woolf, 1974). Therefore, knowledge refinement is to improve that which can be perceived or learned by introducing subtleties or distinctions. This implies not only analysis of existing knowledge but efforts to gradually change that knowledge to a more advanced level.

Knowledge generation and knowledge refinement are the bases of a scientific discipline. Research and theory construction are two major ways of generating or refining knowledge. The major portion of this book has focused on these two approaches. But they are not the only ways of generating or refining knowledge. We will first review what some nurse-authors have said about knowledge generation and refinement. Then we will look at different authors' discussions of ways of knowing. We will conclude by trying to synthesize the various approaches to knowledge generation and refinement with the various ways of knowing. We will offer some suggestions about the functions of the different ways of knowing for knowledge generation and refinement.

DIMENSIONALITY OF THE DISCIPLINE

Ellis (1983) reasoned that empirical science provides answers only to certain questions about nursing. Other questions, such as "What is the meaning of dignity? What does it mean to be compassionate, humane, and caring?" (p. 212), remain to be answered. These are questions that cannot be answered by empirical science. In such matters as these, philosophic inquiry must take the lead. As Ellis saw it, philosophic inquiry is a method of examining meanings in existing knowledge that leads to knowledge refinement. Scientific inquiry, on the other hand, is the search for new knowledge or knowledge generation. In her review of nursing inquiries focused on philosophy, she found four categories or types of knowledge refinement. These were ethics; philosophy of nursing education; concepts, values, and processes; and methodology. Ethics was concerned with the study of morality, judgment, and obligation in nursing. Philosophy of nursing education focused on issues such as commitment and caring and investigations related to beliefs and values in curricula. The concepts, values, and processes inquiries focused on issues such as empathy, health, quality of life, healing, heroism, judgment, and meaning in suffering. The methodological inquiries were very dissimilar in content but all proposed methods for studying nursing. All of the methodological inquiries cautioned against relying on science for all explanations about nursing at the expense of the pervasive values in nursing, such as ideas of humanitarianism, holism, and individualism.

Donaldson and Crowley (1978) argue that nursing as a discipline is bigger than nursing as a science and that nursing's uniqueness is more a function of its perspective than its methods of inquiry. They suggest that three traditional sources of knowledge—science, history, and philosophy—are the most salient for knowledge generation and refinement in nursing. Beckstrand (1978, 1980), in critiquing the notion of practice theory, concluded that even though nursing knowledge was not well articulated, it did exist and could be further developed through the use of the methods of science, ethics, and philosophy. Silva (1977) proposed that all nursing science begins and ends with philosophy. She suggested that the four branches of philosophy—logic, epistomology, metaphysics, and ethics—in addition to intuition and introspection are all useful methods for generating and developing knowledge.

It can be seen from the foregoing discussion that several nurse-authors are thoughtfully considering the generation and refinement of nursing knowledge. It is not surprising that their ideas overlap substantially. Each of the perspectives presented has shown that not all knowledge generation or refinement can or should be derived from empirical science. They have also pointed to the fact that nursing is not a unidimensional discipline but a multidimensional one. They have identified the need for different perspectives in the development of nursing knowledge. They have not, however, gone as far as we need to go in our thinking on this issue. It seems to us that the second or next step in this process is to consider the needs for various types of knowledge in nursing practice and to think about how that knowledge can and should be used within the discipline. Again, viewing our phenomena of interest from different perspectives and viewpoints is critical.

Visintainer's (1986) idea of perceptual maps is very much to the point here. Perceptual maps, she asserts, serve much the same function as topographical maps, weather maps, maps of mineral deposits, and road maps. Each map contains relevant information about some geographic region, but a weather map does not contain information about mineral deposits. In the same way, the knowledge base in nursing may be viewed through perceptual maps. Each perceptual map will provide a slightly different view of the same "region" of knowledge. In fact, it seems to us that using different perceptual maps at different times during knowledge refinement serves several functions. First, using several different perceptual maps will assure a breadth of perspective within the nursing discipline. In the early days of nursing, our knowledge was overbalanced on the side of esthetics, the knowing by doing that is the art of nursing. More recently, the scale has tilted toward "empirical-scientific" knowing.

Second, using different perceptual maps at different times during study of a phenomenon will lead to different and useful insights depending on which map is being used. These insights into the phenomenon would not be available without the guidance of the maps. A more profound understanding of the phenomenon can be acquired in this manner than from using the perspective of one map.

Third, the use of several perceptual maps is useful during decision making prior to developing research programs or planning theory construction. Each map will suggest different questions and different approaches to answering them. This facilitates the generation of new knowledge.

Finally, we believe that using different perceptual maps in clinical practice is also a useful way to develop knowledge. Examining nursing care from several perspectives will give clinicians as well as scholars needed insights into what is effective care in which situations, thus leading to more efficient diagnoses and interventions in practice.

ALTERNATE WAYS OF KNOWING

In this section we will examine two different author's ideas about knowing and try to offer some suggestions about how the different ways of knowing and the perspectives on generating and refining knowledge fit together.

Zbilut (1978) identified four "habits" of thinking: "empiriological-experiential," "empirical-metaphenomenal," "philosophical-metaphenomenal," and "philosophical-transcendental." Empiriological-experiential thinking incorporates personal experience and scientific reasoning and research. Empirical-metaphenomenal thinking has to do with hypotheses, theories, and laws. Philosophical-metaphenomenal thinking has to do with humanness and problems of man's existence in relation to a space-time axis. Finally, philosophical-transcendental thinking focuses on building bridges between formal philosophy and "real world" concerns. Zbilut argues that there are some things that cannot be known without participation in them. Objectivity and observation cannot fully explain how one "knows" another person, for example. Zbilut's four habits of thinking would each generate a different kind of knowing. Knowing about patients in pain from an empiriological-metaphenomenal habit of thinking would be very different from knowing about the same patients from the philosophical-metaphenomenal habit of thinking. The questions raised from each habit of thought and the answers arrived at for those questions will generate different types of knowledge.

From a study of nursing literature, Carper (1978) identified four ways or patterns of knowing in nursing. Her proposed four ways of knowing are empirics, esthetics, personal knowledge, and ethics. Since Carper's ideas have received considerable attention in the literature, we will explain each way of knowing in more detail than Zbilut's.

The first way of knowing is empirics, or the science of nursing. She describes this pattern as empirical, factual, descriptive, and aimed at developing explanations. The link between this pattern of knowing, theory refinement, and theory testing is clear. The bulk of this book has focused on this aspect of knowing.

The second way of knowing is esthetics, or the art of nursing. Esthetics is concerned with expression and with the technical skills of nursing that contribute to the art of practice. An esthetic experience involves the creation and/or appreciation of singular, subjective expressions that resist description in language. Esthetics involves perception, synthesis, and creativity—putting parts together into a whole that is satisfying. Empathy is one action made available through esthetics. The smooth rhythm and skill of an experienced nurse giving an injection might be another. Esthetics are experiences independent of any connection other than their own realities. The esthetic pattern and appreciation of a "whole" may provide insight into a phenomenon that no one has clearly seen before.

The third way of knowing in nursing is the component of personal knowledge. Personal knowledge is concerned with the knowing, encountering, and actualizing of the self. It is not knowing about the self, but simply knowing the self. Personal knowledge is existential in focus, for example, it is concerned with an individual's being and what that individual can become. Nurses who use their personal knowledge in treating clients will view each one as unique and constantly new, and their care will reflect that view.

The fourth way of knowing is ethical knowing. This way of knowing is focused on the "oughts" or "shoulds" of life, the moral obligations we assume. Knowing about morality in nursing goes beyond simply understanding and being guided by norms or codes of ethics for the discipline. It includes all goals and actions that nurses plan and implement in the care of patients. Each goal and each action involves a choice that is made, at least partially, from the nurse's conception of what "ought" to be done, in other words from some value judgment. Carper argues that the ethical way of knowing in nursing requires an understanding of varying philosophical and ethical frameworks for determining what is right or good, or what ought to be done. Not all patients, nor in fact all nurses, use the same frameworks for deciding what is right or good. Moral decision making is potentially very complex, and nurses giving care to patients may find that their own values and beliefs conflict with their patients' values. Carper suggests that moral choices in these cases should be focused on specific actions for specific situations, taking into account the perspective of each participant.

The habits or ways of knowing discussed above have many areas of overlap with the previous authors' ideas about knowledge generation and refinement. Indeed it seems clear that each habit or way of knowing would lend itself to a particular kind of knowledge refinement. For example, the habit of empiriological-experiential thinking and the empirical way of knowing are clearly linked to the methods of empirical science. The habit of philosophical-metaphenomenal thinking and the ethical way of knowing are clearly linked to philosophy and ethics. Each habit of thinking or way of knowing will provide a different view or perspective on any phenomenon of interest.

Meleis (1987) has argued for the need to revise our passion for methodologies, science, and philosophy to allow room for a passion for substance, that is, the "business" of nursing or the domain concepts. She, too, speaks for the need for nurse scientists to use all available methods for generating knowledge to "achieve a range of perceptions, experiences, and meanings."

It seems to us that the ways of knowing and the proposed ways of generating and developing knowledge are like the warp and woof in weaving. Without both, the weaver's fabric is incomplete and full of holes. With both on the loom, the fabric is strong and the patterns and colors are clear and beautiful. But the patterns and colors in the fabric will be different depending on the perspective of the individual weaver. In the same way, the ways of knowing and the different methods of generating and developing knowledge used together will provide a strong base fabric of knowledge in nursing. The differing perspectives of different scientists will provide richness and depth to the patterns that are identified.

One example of this type of study comes immediately to mind. Woods's studies of the experiences of perimenstrual symptoms in women have used several perspectives to obtain a whole picture of the phenomenon. Her methods have ranged from detailed microanalysis of nutritional patterns to investigating the impact of poverty and feminine socialization on women experiencing perimenstrual symptoms (Woods et al., 1982; Woods et al., 1987; Woods, 1987). By using various research methods, both quantitative and qualitative, and by asking questions from several perspectives, Woods and her colleagues have made a substantial contribution to nursing's knowledge about the phenomenon of menstruation and the events surrounding it.

We think it is imperative for nurse scholars to use all the different percepual maps and ways of knowing to develop the knowledge base of our discipline, and for caring, responsible practice. Finally, it is important that we keep in mind that in a practice discipline such as nursing, knowledge for knowledge's sake is useful, but knowledge for practice is paramount.

REFERENCES

Beckstrand J: The need for a practice theory as indicated by the knowledge used in the conduct of practice. Res Nurs and Health 1(4): 175–179, 1978.
Beckstrand J: A critique of several conceptions of practice theory in nursing. Res Nurs and Health 3: 69–79, 1980.
Carper BA: Fundamental patterns of knowing in nursing. Adv Nurs Sci 1(1): 13–23, 1978.
Donaldson SK, Crowley DM: The discipline of nursing. Nurs Outlook 26(2): 113–120, 1978.
Ellis R: Philosophic inquiry. In (HH Werley & JJ Fitzpatrick, eds.), Annual Rev Nurs Res 1: 211–228, 1983.
Halsey WD (ed.): Macmillan Contemporary Dictionary. New York: Macmillan, 1979.
Meleis AN: ReVisions in knowledge development: A passion for substance. Schol Inquiry for Nurs Prac 1(1): 5–19, 1987.
Silva MC: Philosophy, science, theory: Interrelationships and implications for nursing research. Image 9(3): 59–63, 1977.
Visintainer MA: The nature of knowledge and theory in nursing. Image 18(2): 32–38, 1986.
Woods NF: Response: Early morning musings on the passion for substance. Schol Inquiry for Nurs Prac 1(1): 25–28, 1987.
Woods NF, Lenz M, Mitchell E, Taylor D, Lee K, and Barash N: Perimenstrual symptoms, social environment, socialization, health practices, and health status. Final Report to the National Center for Nursing Research, USPHS, 1987.
Woods NF, Most A, Dery G: Prevalence of perimenstrual symptoms. Amer J of Pub Health 72(11): 1257–1264, 1982.
Woolf HB: Webster's New Collegiate Dictionary. Springfield, Mass.: G & C Merriam, 1974.
Zbilut JP: Epistemologic constraints to the development of a theory in nursing. Nurs Res 27: 128–129, 1978.

Index

Italicized letters following page numbers indicate tables (*t*) and figures (*f*).

Italicized letters following page numbers indicate tables (*t*) and figures (*f*).

Italicized letters following page numbers indicate tables (*t*) and figures (*f*).

Italicized letters following page numbers indicate tables (*t*) and figures (*f*).

Italicized letters following page numbers indicate tables (*t*) and figures (*f*).

Italicized letters following page numbers indicate tables (*t*) and figures (*f*).